To Beth,

Remember,
Fiber is your Friend
+ attitude is
everything :)

Hugs, + insulin,
Lauren

TYPE
ONE
DETERMINATION

**Transforming type 1 diabetes
through personal experience, scientific evidence,
and a dash of disobedience**

LAUREN PLUNKETT

ISBN-13: 978-1-63489-473-9

Library of Congress Catalog Number has been applied for.
Printed in the United States of America
First Printing: 2021

25 24 23 22 21   5 4 3 2 1

Cover design by Michael Berglund
Interior design by Patrick Maloney

Wise Ink Creative Publishing
807 Broadway St NE
Suite 46
Minneapolis, MN, 55413

I am a registered dietitian with type 1 diabetes. I wrote this book to help my patients, and people like them, live happier, fuller lives. This book should be used to supplement, rather than replace, the advice of your doctor or other licensed health professional. Please see your healthcare provider before beginning any new health program or treatment.

This publication is written and published to provide accurate and authoritative information relevant to the subject matter presented. All efforts have been made to assure the accuracy of the information contained in this book as of the date of publication.

I dedicate this book to my parents for always supporting and believing in their free-spirited boomerang child.

"It is not the strongest of the species that survive,
nor the most intelligent,
but the one most responsive to change."
—Leon C. Megginson

TABLE OF CONTENTS

An Introduction to Building Your Scientific Badassery......... 1

A COMEBACK STORY
1. Cola and Candy Bars 7
2. Going Mental 19
3. The Rebellion Begins 30
4. Shipwrecked on Diabetes Island...................... 42
5. Feeding the Disease... 52
6. The Cornerstones.. 64
7. Break the Wheel 77
8. Move the Needle... 89
9. Language and Attitude..................................... 94

NUTRITION
Nutrition Knowledge....................................... 107
History of Nutrition in Diabetes....................... 116
Fiber 124
Diet Culture and Diabetes 134
Modern Challenges.. 141
Eating with Eyes Open 144

EXERCISE
Exercise Knowledge 163
Exercise Protocol.. 170
Mental Toughness... 182
Metabolism, Calories, and Protein 187
Carbohydrate Restrictions in Athletes 195
Embrace the Contrasts..................................... 203

Blood Glucose Conversion Chart....................... 209
Educational and Motivational Resources 210
Outro 211
Acknowledgments.. 212
Notes 215

AN INTRODUCTION TO BUILDING YOUR SCIENTIFIC BADASSERY

Chronic disease can be a teacher—
the type that tells you to make good decisions when you leave in
the morning and to come home smarter at the end of the day

I HAVE NO IDEA what it's like not to inject a needle into my body every couple of hours, nor do I know how it feels to eat without analyzing my food. I am completely dependent on the medical technology that keeps me alive, and even the slightest change in routine can completely restructure my day. The concept of leaving the house without food and a blood sugar monitor is entirely unknown. But I'm not complaining. What comes with great difficulty provides the opportunity to grow as a person capable of many things—including the mental fortitude of a fighter.

I know how it feels to be identified as a medical-record number and looked at like a pitiful danger to myself. As a patient in the healthcare system for over half my life, my worth has been determined by measurements in my blood—the most authentic substance flowing within.

From the beginning, I was given permission to set the bar low and accept that struggling through a mediocre existence was as good as it would ever get. *Healthy* would never be my adjective.

I used to be scared of a lot of stuff: bridges, the dark, exercise, tequila—anything I couldn't control or that could hinder my ability to read my body from the inside out. I used to feel limited by my fears, but I wasn't put on this planet to get pushed around by anybody, or anything, just because my body isn't perfect. In fact, imperfection is an astounding gift.

It took fifteen years of living with type 1 diabetes (T1D), dozens of visits with doctors and educators, five different colleges, and buckets of angry tears before I understood that I was capable of being healthy. The catch was, I had to believe it for myself.

Degrading words spoken with indifference by doctors and dietitians turned me from a carefree kid into an angry little girl with big responsibilities. The bad experiences mounted with frustration in my teenage years, but as a young adult, my feelings about healthcare expanded. I found myself consumed by the damage that medical professionals and uninformed people can do with insensitive language and inadequate advice.

Depending on the education protocol and teaching method presented at diagnosis, it may appear that life with diabetes is supposed to be lived a certain way to prevent complications. The outside world may look upon everyone with diabetes as either unhealthy or unfortunate. I felt that carrying around a blood sugar monitor everywhere I went had stamped "disease" to my forehead for all to see and judge. On the inside, I concealed a loaded lunch box of shame, confusion, and anger, trying to force myself to adhere to regulated expectations.

Living with diabetes is never just a narrow scope of rules about food, insulin, and exercise, but defined by multiple layers of emotions, impacting mental health, self-confidence, and hope for the future.

Since the discovery and administration of insulin just over one hundred years ago, treatment has focused on a nutrition protocol that demands carbohydrate restriction to prevent unhealthy blood sugar levels. Though scientific evidence has evolved, the message that carbs continue to be the problem lives on through methods of extreme control. When rigid methods don't work, a patient with diabetes is often labeled as noncompliant rather than presented with a different path of treatment—one that is personal, focuses on the whole person, and provides tools to advance self-sufficient skills.

As for me, "noncompliant" may as well have been tattooed across my face.

Barreling through the hormonal apocalypse into young adulthood was like living in the eye of a hurricane. There was only one way to live with T1D that I knew of, and I was bad at it, even though I was trying. Not meeting expectations translated into failure as I lost myself within the system of diabetes management. I felt trapped and constricted by a disease that I didn't completely understand, while trying to discover myself at the same time. This perfect storm was a tragedy, but through the struggle I would learn what I needed to emerge undefeated.

What started as an adventure in staying alive became a mission in turning *why*s into wisdom.

Learning how to live a meaningful life, as opposed to stumbling around like a hungry zombie on a sugar high, begins with questions.

Why don't I understand insulin better?

Why do I spend so much time feeling angry?

Why are nutrition and exercise so complicated—*why, dammit, why?!*

If you're nodding your head in agreement, *I got you, friend.*

The cornerstones of diabetes—glucose, insulin, exercise, and nutrition—have guided me through life, but I didn't always know how important the relationship is between the cornerstones and my values. Pushing diabetes away only kept the wheel of angry unhappiness spinning wildly as I struggled to hold on. For years, I wasted time fighting a losing battle as an opposing force, until I understood how to interact with my body in partnership with scientific evidence. Discovering the health benefits of plant-based nutrition sparked my curiosity as I uncovered the interconnection of chronic disease to all the systems of the body, and how eating fewer animal products and more plants could change the health of the world.

As a lifelong student of diabetes with knowledge of the patient experience, I was determined to become the person I needed most. The one-way perspective of diabetes management never produced results, and I woke up realizing that I had to become an expert. Accepting that diabetes was a part of me, but not all of me, adjusted my identity, making space to align my values with goal-oriented decisions.

I developed a warrior's mindset while I was under construction, acquiring a skill set and knowledge bank that propelled me forward as a force for change. Driven by everything I saw wrong with diabetes education, I became a professional who can talk the talk as a living example. I've used my experiences to build a healthier foundation for myself that can be replicated for others with evidence that, through diabetes, we can thrive on knowledge, courage, and ironlike determination.

We may feel limited by diabetes at times, but we do not have to suffer, endure poor treatment, or let negativity direct our attitude. Diabetes, in particular, can be the mark of a new beginning that jump-starts a healthier perspective on life with a fresh set of choices. We can let disease determine our actions and attitude, or we can be daring and embrace it. By using diabetes to understand ourselves better, we become empowered.

My personal and professional obligation as part of a worldwide diabetes community is to be clear about who we are, what we need, and what we can do.

In addition, I'm passing on the responsibility to you, my reader, to pay your knowledge forward, sharing in the common goal of elevating all those living with diabetes.

So, turn the page and take a walk with me back to the beginning . . .

PART ONE

A COMEBACK STORY

From Diagnosed to
Downright Determined

1

COLA AND CANDY BARS

I wasn't supposed to make it to my twelfth birthday

OCTOBER 1993. MINNESOTA. Slightly above freezing.
"Lauren, are you ready?!" Mom, high pitched from the kitchen. "We've got to leave for your appointment. Dad's coming too."

"Hold on! I gotta pee." Again.

Less than ten minutes later, I urgently landed on the toilet at our family practice clinic.

We were all lucky the bathroom was vacant. The decorative waiting room ficus sat in an oversized pot, and I wasn't afraid to squat in it.

It wasn't a secret to anyone who spent more than a few minutes in the same room with me that something was off. Within a few months I had developed an insatiable thirst, had cottonmouth between drinks, and urgently needed to urinate often. Sugar was my one true love that I craved endlessly, the only thing powering my body, but with zero energy to show for it.

My sunken eyes were clear evidence of metabolic meltdown, and even as I drank more Coke than water, I became frail from weight loss.

Coincidentally, my parents happened to meet a couple with a daughter who had recently been diagnosed with something I was about to have in common with her. They described similar symptoms prior to diagnosis, and the next thing I knew, I had an appointment to see a doctor.

The universe works in mysterious ways when we're looking for answers.

After this foretelling conversation, my parents were on me like white on rice. Every afternoon when I came home from school, I devoured a full-size candy bar and washed it down with a can of soda. The calories meant nothing. All the while, I was slowly wasting away. This had been my afternoon snack for several months, and I didn't see anything wrong with it.

In fact, I had it made as a chunky kid, losing weight while eating chocolate bars.

"ALL RIGHT, I'M back." After my third trip to the bathroom.

I was weighed and directed toward an exam room where Mom and Dad were already talking with the doctor. I hopped up on the exam table, preparing to answer questions by licking my lips and peeling my tongue off the roof of my mouth, which was bone dry again.

The worried look my parents shared indicated that this exam was going to be different from what I'd known. Before we left the mountains of the West for the rolling hills of Minnesota, I had breathing problems that suddenly stopped. With the change in environment and altitude, I no longer needed asthma medication or the occasional nebulizer. My old pediatrician had prescribed every new medication that walked into his office to see if it would open up my airways. By the time we arrived in Minnesota, I had already experimented with dozens of different pharmaceutical compounds before I was ten years old.

The exam began on a papered table with the basic inspections: ears, eyes, throat, reflexes, and other nonverbal observations. So far, all normal, but it got weird when the doctor took a whiff of my breath.

What's this? C'mon, I brushed!

Then I got my finger stabbed for the first time ever. Not cool. That poker thing was vicious.

Disposable finger-stick devices are comparable in comfort to the iron maiden of the Dark Ages.

. . . and something I would have to get used to.

My new doctor set in motion a lifequake that changed everything about my future.

I liked her straight, shoulder-length black hair, which made me think of Cleopatra. She wore bright red lipstick and had a gentle manner. She was quirky for a primary care physician, and I liked that too. Every checkup before this one had been uneventful, so why wouldn't today be the same?

"I'm going to run this, and I'll be back shortly," Dr. Cleopatra said with a telling, sympathetic smile.

Something was up. Hopefully, whatever she was running wouldn't take long. I had to pee, and I needed a Coke.

"Mom, I'm really thirsty. Can I get some water?" ·

I couldn't sit there one minute longer without emptying my bladder and slurping at the water fountain like a Labrador. I was so thirsty, and my mouth felt like I had been chewing on insulation-flavored gum.

I didn't know much, but I did know it wasn't right that I woke up several times a night to pee and drink out of the faucet. It was annoying and a little embarrassing. Yet, at eleven years old, I had recently become more aware of what my body looked like compared to other girls my age. I was new in town the year before, and I liked being from another place, but I didn't want to stand out for the wrong reasons. I was preparing to start sixth grade baby fat–free, and I was looking super lean.

Being different was cool, but I didn't want to be weird.

I especially didn't want to be fat. *What could be worse?*

I had a bit of a junk food problem prior to getting sick. Losing weight while eating candy bars was a fat kid's winning Powerball ticket. While my body was starting to deteriorate, I discovered that I could eat anything and wake up lighter the next day. Maybe I was one of the lucky girls who could eat whatever she wanted and be skinny, I thought.

The changes happened very fast, and I wasn't going to fix the problem on my own. The scariest symptom of all was that I was getting used to how terrible I felt.

I had been in sixth grade about one month when I landed in the exam room. All I was focused on was my last year of elementary school and solidifying my place in the social hierarchy of gal pals. Evidently, there were only two options in this town: sporty and good at it, or quit while you're ahead. I'd have to pick a lucky number and try out for something. It was that, or be weird. Because the opinions of others were important, and I wanted to be liked.

It was impossible to know what the trigger was that caused my body to attack itself, and I didn't want to admit that I felt like I was dying. I was way too tired to do my favorite things, like draw and annoy my dad by making bike-tire tracks through his freshly mowed lawn. No matter how much I wanted to fit in, trying out for a fall sport was totally out of the question. Not only was my body a wreck, but my mind was full of fog, and my reactions were ultra slow. Cluelessly falling apart at the seams, all I could do was watch TV, drink, and pee.

Just a few minutes had passed when Dr. Cleopatra quietly entered the room to deliver the historic blow. Words were spoken in a fragile tone, but it was tense, as if we'd all burst into a million water droplets. The only words I remember came from the doc and are frozen in my memory like a Polaroid picture: "Based on her signs and symptoms . . . this is diabetes."

Have I fallen into a vortex? Time suddenly warped into a dimension like being on a climbing roller coaster that suddenly pauses at the pinnacle of fear and adrenaline before pitching over the edge. My bladder was maxed out again, and I couldn't hold back the tears. My body was liquified. I was crying about something I knew nothing about, but my parents had prepared themselves. All I could do was sit there in tearful confusion.

I leaned my failing, sugar-filled body against my dad and realized the candy bars would have to go. It was too good to be true anyway.

The truth was, I was too full of something much more dangerous than urine and sugar to stay alive. My body was using an acidic by-product of body fat in the form of large ketones to keep my organs functioning, and if this was left untreated, I would not survive. This state of metabolic mayhem is called diabetic ketoacidosis, or DKA, a result of dehydration and high amounts of glucose, or sugar, in the blood.

DKA can be thought of as the signature of new-onset type 1 diabetes. When the pancreas does not produce enough insulin, a hormone that shuttles glucose to cells, energy plummets. We cannot function without a constant supply of glucose entering cells, but the body is smart enough to provide a short-term solution by producing ketones.

> Glucose is the primary fuel source from head to toe. Nutrients, including glucose, travel through the blood to every organ and, of particular importance, the brain. Nutrient deficiencies along with muscle and tissue loss are a result of DKA and relying on ketones for fuel. This demonstrates why ketosis is an adaptation process not meant for long-term use. In the absence of insulin, blood sugar remains at a dangerously high level with nutrient depletion, and blood vessels become stressed in places like the eyes, heart, and brain.

I was fading to nothing and craving sugar in epic proportions because my body was eating itself alive to prevent a complete systemic meltdown. My cells were starving due to a lack of nourishment, while the glucose in my blood continued to elevate each time I ate because it had nowhere else to go. Evidently, I was down to my last days as an insulin maker, while I continued to get thinner and sicker in its absence.

I was still alive, but barely.

To survive this diagnosis, I would need fluid and electrolytes to restore my blood pH level to resolve the DKA, followed by a hearty replenishment of nutrients.

Bye-Bye, Beta Cells

I was officially living with type 1 diabetes now.
Still kicking, but confused as ever.

Doctor Cleopatra urged my parents to immediately check me into Children's Hospital, where I was admitted for the next three nights. My memory of the hospital stay is blurry—like trying to see out a frosted window. I knew my surroundings, but I didn't know what was happening.

Distinctly, I remember the feeling of coming back to life as my brain processed the current events. Bright-colored stars on the walls, animal-shaped stickers, and kid-themed common areas. Except for the bloody red intravenous catheter on top of my right hand, everything was white in my room, where the disease was concealed.

When I started feeling better, the first movie I watched was *Aladdin*.

"A whole new world, a dazzling place I never knew . . ." How true this was.

There was always a new sympathetic face apologizing for drawing blood from my small, malnourished hand. The catheter ached from the moment it was placed and with each draw that occurred every hour, on the hour, for three nights. I remember thinking, *Blood smells warm,* as my eyes watered and I pretended not to feel pain.

The constant flow of observers entering my room got old fast. But after the first night, my one job was simple: *EAT.*

I was renewed by the feeling of food working inside of me again. The need to feed was such a strong urge that it outweighed the discomfort from insulin injections. Yet, eating six times each day wasn't appealing. Since when was I supposed to eat *this* much food?

Day by day, the replenishment of insulin brought me back into my body, but the clarity brought awareness of my surroundings and suspicion of the professionals feeling sorry for me. If anyone had the power to build my confidence, it would be the people who knew diabetes before it found me. I didn't like the sorry looks of pity, nor did I think that everyone wearing a hospital badge deserved my trust. *Stop acting like my life is going to suck.*

On the second day, my parents and I sat for Insulin Dosing and Carb Counting 101, but my mind was elsewhere; every second I endured was one moment closer to going home. Though I was still recovering, I pushed myself through lessons, hoping the medical staff would send me home the second I proved capable of the basics. Sure enough, I became a finger-poking professional, and I wasn't afraid of injections either. Insulin and I were fast friends.

This was also the first time I heard the words *carbohydrate* and *grams* used to describe food. Counting carbs was a big deal, and I wasn't allowed to eat until a nurse determined how many grams of carbs were in my meals. Every fifteen grams of carbs equaled one unit of insulin drawn up and injected into my thigh.

The lessons I was beginning to learn about insulin involved firm rules that positioned diabetes as a rigid responsibility, but I felt like everything would get better once I got home.

I got this, now go away. I just wanted to leave, but there was so much my parents and I were tasked with doing. The teaching was a combination of instruction and fear; there were rules and hard lines that had to be followed. I would not be allowed to join the military or become a pilot. Fine. I had been thinking about studying sea turtles anyway.

There was a constant undertone of "There could be a cure tomorrow" and "Don't lose hope."

Maybe my parents needed to hear that, but I hated it. *Why am I going through all of this if we should pretend that diabetes could be gone tomorrow?*

Eventually I made it home, and with time, my parents and I got into the groove of our new diabetes routine. Fear was not a factor while we did what we had to do. We were superadapters by making it our own and rolling with the challenge. We took it one day at a time, and life was normal again, but it came with new challenges for me internally. Food was the answer to my suffering, and I was ravenous. Within a short period of time, it was evident that curbing my appetite was like trying to control a fire-breathing dragon.

How long had it been since I absorbed any food?

Nutrients are the key to restoring the body back to health when T1D is diagnosed. When the body isn't producing enough insulin, nutrients from food are not absorbed properly because the body is in a state of metabolic starvation. To prevent further damage, the solution is to inject insulin to better absorb vitamins, minerals, and fluid.

As I ate, I could feel my eyes focusing better, warmth at the surface of my skin; I was alive in a way that I had forgotten the feeling of. My body had been flushing out vitality for who knows how long, while the source of energy I desperately needed, glucose, was trapped in my bloodstream. I was undernourished even though I had been eating plenty of calories up until the day I was diagnosed.

For a kid approaching puberty, this was the time to start eating well, but I had no idea that my new role would demand so much from me. My sixth-grade priorities took a major shift away from social status and toward grown-up-level responsibilities. I had no sense of what I would have to endure for the next decade before waking up and completely changing my path in life.

For the rest of the school year, my thoughts were occupied with a way of living that was a lot more challenging than the way my friends got to live. I had the guts to stick a needle in my body without hesitation before I turned twelve, for crying out loud! My skills were special. I simply had to live in the moment and accept that among my new daily tasks were finger sticks, injections, and bucking up.

I recognize now that being diagnosed was my second chance at life, and that I did nothing wrong in my first eleven years on earth to deserve this disease—but for some reason, *it deserved me*, and someday, I would challenge the way people think about life with disease.

Unfortunately, standard methods in place to help me survive were not designed to help me understand my feelings. The highest expectation for me was to conform and make do with diabetes, secondary only to *don't get dead*. It was as if I were supposed to settle on misfortune and recite a mantra, wishing for a cure every day instead of stepping up to the plate.

Was I supposed to settle as the world's okay-est diabetic? *I think not.*

Like a true eleven-year-old, I put up some resistance to the rules and tasks, but I decided to accept T1D as something I would live with forever. My only choice was to accept diabetes and commit to the new duties of staying alive. Otherwise, how would I ever see the bright side of life again?

Brace Yourself

My time was quietly spent in shame, frustration, and anger for years after I was diagnosed with T1D, as the wrecking ball that is puberty approached. My teenage body was conflicted, my mental health was unstable, and my temper was barely containable once the fuse was lit.

I was extremely private underneath the shame in my sugared-up veins, as the perpetual wheel of diabetes responsibilities turned in my mind. Every day began and ended with a blood sugar check. The number displayed by the monitor determined my attitude for the next several hours, until I checked again. While I was awake, my emotions ran the gauntlet between finger sticks. While I was asleep, my subconscious worried about my blood sugar going low the next day, eating too much, and gaining weight.

I tried not to show my sour feelings because I hated people asking how I was. Teenage insecurity mixed with a dash of anger, plus an organ that didn't fully function, often led to a day concluding with a meltdown. *How's that for teenage angst?*

I gained weight rapidly, my complexion was blemished, and I had braces and then glasses. *Simply horrifying.* Taking part in small talk was like being trapped in an elevator with a fart.

"How is school?" or "What have you been up to this summer?" were not questions I wanted to answer. The honest reply: "Oh, the usual. Craving sugar, watching my body awkwardly grow, and popping zits on the daily, but *how are you?*"

My whole world revolved around insulin, test strips, and food. In my honest opinion, I was at liberty to be outrageously pissed.

I had a mind of my own and a tongue like a razor blade, which wasn't exactly a friend maker. From a young age, I was taught not to take any crap from anybody, and if something went really wrong, "Call your brothers" was Dad's order.

The influence of two older brothers and a military-officer father spiced up disease management rather creatively. Dad had a way of establishing some serious rules about conduct and decision-making that'll stick with a kid. I needed exceptional life skills beyond the basics. If there's one thing I know about my dad, it's that it's not wise to make him worry, so I took his lessons seriously. As a result, I matured fast and developed a quick wit that kept me in better company most of the time.

Diabetes forced me to act like an adult when it came to reading a situation and making smart decisions, because my life literally depended on my ability to not accidentally kill myself. Besides, the last thing I needed was to get busted by my dad for making bad choices. Most importantly, I didn't want to let him down. He invested a lot of time into raising a proper lady who made the right choices, while having the skills to throw a punch if she had to.

Because I had more responsibility than other kids my age, my thoughts were occupied with more important things than gossip. Did I think I was better than everybody else? Kind of. Better in the way that I knew if I partied hard, did drugs, or got drunk, bad judgment could lead to the last decision I ever made.

I was particularly alert to the inconsiderate things that came out of my classmates' mouths, and I didn't want any part of it. Some of them seemed to enjoy being passively mean, as if saying "Just kidding" after calling somebody stupid erased their intention. Fearing that I might lose control of my tongue if I got mad, my solution was to skip social gatherings to avoid drawing attention to my diabetes.

On the outside, I looked tough and confident, but on the inside, I was as fragile as cotton candy. There wasn't anything my peers could say about me that I wasn't already aware of. In my mind, I wasn't athletic enough, smart enough, or pretty enough. All I wanted was to be the best at one thing to take the attention off my diabetes. *Surely, excellence should come effortlessly in some area to compensate for all these injections?*

As the years went on, it became utterly evident that "easy" was never going to be an option for me. I would always be surrounded by people with fully functioning pancreases, while I was stuck living in a damaged body. Every three months, I was required to check in at the diabetes clinic to be analyzed for irreparable damage due to poor control. I felt like a car in the shop that continuously had its check-engine light on, when all I ever got was an oil change.

Attention fell on the same issues that had a quick fix, while the persistent problems remained, burrowing deeper into the root of who I was becoming.

2

GOING MENTAL

The relationship between disease and emotions is undeniable

INSULIN HELPED NOURISH my body back to health, but that came with a new challenge. I was gaining weight faster than a mouse in a Twinkie factory. Puberty was knocking, and I had absolutely no idea how to manage my relentless sugar cravings, or balance insulin and exercise. There were so many factors to consider, and I tried doing what I was told, but diabetes isn't the most predictable friend.

The effort I put forth was not making me look good, and I paid for it in self-worth. Doctors tossed around terms like *normal, noncompliant,* and *poorly controlled* to describe my body. I had to prove my daily effort through a blood test. *Did I really just get called an "uncontrolled diabetic"? Hey, I'm standing right here, and I'm not dead yet! Does this look easy to you?*

I became highly sensitive to words that were frequently used to describe me, and I took them personally.

The turmoil that boiled inside of me was toxic. Based on my lab results, the experts might say that I was at risk of losing a limb, my eyesight, or a kidney. I never knew how future-crushing the conversation would be at any given appointment. In this atmosphere, hope and self-sufficiency were tied up in a straitjacket and banished to a dark corner.

The pediatric education system for diabetes is directed toward parents who need the skills to safely deliver medications, and that's understandable. Parents must be capable of carrying out the basics of diabetes care for their children with T1D. The problem is, the clinic is not a school that teaches *kids* how to leverage their disease into a skill set they can use to build strength, character, and courage. The numbers determined my worth, and the topics on the clipboard weren't about me, but about diabetes. Who I was, how I felt, and what I was struggling with in my heart and head held no space on the agenda. Nor did I want to contribute. Every time I thought it might get better, I returned home a little more broken.

However, I had a pretty good teacher at home, and I would not be allowed to pout my way through life. There wasn't anything in this world, not even diabetes, that could get between me and my dad's school of character-building life lessons.

Commander Plunkett

Diagnosis causes a person to grow up fast and face responsibilities. I went from playing with Barbies and pretending I was a princess to drawing up a syringe and giving myself multiple insulin injections daily.

Diabetes brought a seriousness into my soul, but that didn't erase the person I was before this second chance at life. My new responsibilities added to the high expectations that my dad, a retired navy commander, already had planned. If the doctors treated me like a dysfunctional child, at home, Dad showed me that I was never less than capable.

The yard was a big deal when we moved into our Minnesota house. Half the yard was in the woods, but that didn't stop my dad from twitching every time a leaf lay to rest on his groomed lawn. He'd have that Clint Eastwood look of Wild West determination on his face, scanning the yard from side to side as he pulled his work gloves on nice and tight.

Remember, tomorrow is promised to no one. Like Clint said.

My dad was the fastest rake slinger east of the Mississippi River. I would stare out my bedroom window, wishing the yard were full of palm trees, as my dad unloaded his lawn gear, including a gigantic blue tarp, from the garage. *Stupid blue tarp*, I'd think. I can't imagine what the neighbors thought. Civilized people hired a crew for what went down on our lot.

Dad's weekend routine was as follows:

1. Let the dog out. Get the paper. Make coffee. Deliver a cup to Mom while she's still in bed.
2. Load up the six-disc CD changer. First up: B.B. King.
3. Thunderously walk through the house shouting lyrics.
4. Propose breakfast ideas to Mom as she shuffles into the kitchen for more coffee.
5. Choose waffles. Sort the paper. Sing louder.
6. Wake up the child. "Wake up, Baby, it's morning time!" Aggressively flick on the bedroom light and rub stubble against the child's cheek, pulling the pillow out from under the child's head and tossing it across the room.
7. Thunderously walk back to the kitchen shouting, "Second attempt won't be so nice!"

My childhood friends liked him better than they liked me. But to a teenage daughter, a dad is just another annoying dude.

All-you-can-eat waffle breakfast, despite the sugar-free syrup, typically meant high blood sugar, but not when the inevitable "leaf weekend" was upon me. I didn't know how to avoid going low, so I practiced the not-so-smart method for physical activity that anyone with T1D would understand: I allowed my blood sugar to get really high, so I had a head start before it dropped too low. I burned blood sugar fast when I went to war on a leaf pile and then dragged the stupid tarp full of leaves into the woods to cast off. As fate would have it, I would feel the symptoms of a low within the hour.

Ha-HAA! I thought. *This is my out. I can pull the diabetes card and get out of this leaf-athon to treat myself inside the house.*

"DAAAD!" I screamed as loud as I could. "I'm low and I'm going in!"

He looked up, squinted like Clint, and said, "Well, get yourself a juice box and come right back out. We're not done, and you're not a sissy."

The first time I used a swear word was probably at a time like this. Dad cut no slack. Not for diabetes. Never for being a girl.

Mentally, Dad challenged me to read, be curious, and learn something new every day. There was always something to get up early for, or a story that Dad wanted to tell. He could have us howling so hard with laughter at the dinner table that it took hours to eat.

My brothers and I grew up to share similar work ethics, and when we remind Dad about certain arduous events, his usual reply is, "I don't remember it quite like that, but you turned out okay, didn't ya?"

Dad challenged me because I would always be challenged by life. He encouraged me to build the character of a strong woman who values responsibility, and if I was going to live well, I couldn't quit when things got hard. Diabetes wasn't an excuse then, nor is it an excuse now.

Some of us grow up to be exactly what we wanted to be when we were kids. Lucky ducks get it that easy. The rest of us have to wait tables, take odd jobs, go to college twice, and work our way from the bottom before the tide turns in our favor. I'm thankful that my parents treated me like I deserved to be treated: as a member of the family, no different than any other leaf that fell from the tree.

Brain Power

The commander's expectations were one thing to aim for, but internally, there was good reason to take my health seriously. From head to toe, diabetes makes its presence known. An important organ to consider that isn't often spoken of in diabetes care happens to be the one that requires the most nutrition.

Our demanding human brain has evolved to require a lot of oxygen, along with 20 percent of available blood flow and 20 percent of available glucose, even though it accounts for only 2 percent of body weight! This disproportion in weight to energy requirements leads to a high demand for nutrient flow to the brain, and potential for deficiencies.[1]

Nutrient deficiency can lead to dysfunction in many ways. Severe hypoglycemia, or chronically low blood sugars, can be dangerous to the brain, which is sensitive to extreme changes in blood sugar.

Ketones can act as a substitute under conditions of starvation, as we learned about DKA, but there is nothing quite like glucose. When it comes to nutrients and blood sugar, the flow of glucose to the brain is, without argument, a physiological requirement—preferably provided by healthy sources of carbohydrates, and less from added sugars.

Refined, fast-acting sugar plays an enormous role in the development and progression of cognitive impairment, including Alzheimer's disease, depression, and anxiety, by altering brain chemistry. Fast-acting refined sugar is the ultimate stimulant that lights up brain activity.[2]

Living with T1D provides a unique perspective on how fast-acting sugar can be difficult and uncomfortable for the body to process. Dosing insulin and using a continuous glucose monitor gives us real-time proof of how quickly we must act to avoid drastic fluctuations. In another light, if you are an endurance athlete, fast-acting sugar takes on a performance role to provide rapid, sustainable energy to continue working at the same pace. Taking in loads of fast-acting sugar without putting it to immediate use causes stress and cellular damage over time.

Our diets have changed so much with evolution and lifestyle that functioning today on regular hits of fast-acting sugar is commonplace. In fact, it's a downright addiction that many people struggle to avoid, while our brain, arteries, cells, and metabolism become overwhelmed without warning—the perfect setting for the development of chronic disease. Improving brain function and preventive healthcare work hand in hand.

Type 2 diabetes is marked by insulin resistance: when cells struggle to uptake glucose from the blood to use for energy. Insulin is available to transport glucose to cells, but when cells struggle to take in glucose fast enough, it accumulates in the bloodstream, causing hyperglycemia. Insulin resistance is also caused by fatty particles that build up in muscle cells, primarily from food sources of saturated fat.[3]

In type 1 diabetes, the overeating of high-calorie foods with saturated fat that results in weight gain is likely to cause insulin resistance. In the brain, insulin resistance causes a lack of glucose to brain cells that are known as neurons. Damaged cell structures impair communication between neurons, while plaques form from proteins that would normally be degraded and removed. High added-sugar consumption, insulin resistance, and the formation of plaques lead to cognitive decline.[4]

Diabetes increases risk of Alzheimer's disease and dementia. Early age of onset (five to seven years old), repeated episodes of severely low blood sugars, and duration of time with blood sugars out of range are associated risk factors. But this does not mean people with diabetes are doomed for cognitive decline.[5] The best immediate action for people with diabetes to take is to know the risk factors that may be contributing to insulin resistance.

Too many lows during the night, spending less than 70 percent of the time with blood sugar in range, eating large portions of saturated fat, and not enough whole grains, vegetables, beans, and fruit are controllable risk factors at the top of a long-term healthy agenda. Nourishment supports the highest level of functioning for the brain as the home for memories, thoughts, and intelligence. (To back up your brain with nutrition, see part 2).

Brain health is paramount for a full, healthy life—with or without diabetes. Mental health describes a feeling, whereas the brain is an organ that needs preserving. The way we feel about ourselves impacts the state of our health, and the relationship between disease and emotions is undeniable. When we allow ourselves to accept that burnout or stress affects our quality of life, we take up the opportunity to do something about it and move forward with a strategy.

Falling Off the Road

Opportunities for preventive health education or weight-loss counseling with kids are often skimmed over or put off for another time. Yet parents need to hear this. The prevalence of overweight kids with T1D is estimated at 22 percent,[6] and kids that could benefit from learning healthy habits are usually following the lead of someone at home.

Advanced topics like sports nutrition require special interest that often extends beyond the basic education that clinics usually deliver. To advance skills, it's up to the person with diabetes to ask for individualized education tailored to their specific needs or to find that information elsewhere.

During standard appointments, medical staff will pull data off devices, collect your written log (if you didn't "accidentally" forget it), hand over a questionnaire, and maybe give a sticker or high five. Meeting the doctor includes the standard head-to-toe checkpoints plus a look at injection sites and fingertips before delivering the latest A1c result.

This is where the separation between a human being and a diabetes robot came in for me. A1c was the kingpin that demonstrated how "good" I was doing. My A1c indicated that I wasn't doing very well, but I inched closer to terrible each year, with a nearly double-digit A1c percentage.

Hemoglobin A1c (HbA1c or A1c) is a measurement of blood glucose levels over two to three months.

- Hemoglobin is a protein inside red blood cells that carries oxygen to tissues.

- Glucose attaches to hemoglobin, and it can be measured; this is the A1c test.

- A1c indicates the average glucose level over two to three months as a percentage.

- People without diabetes have an A1c less than 5.7 percent.

- A1c of 5.7–6.4 percent is called prediabetes.

- People are diagnosed with diabetes when A1c is 6.5 percent or higher, as the struggle for cells to take in glucose increases.

- Maintaining A1c at 7 percent or lower decreases the risk of complication over time. To understand A1c better, visualize cells layered in clothing made from sugar:

  - People without diabetes have cells wearing the lightest layers.

  - People with diabetes have cells dressed in anything from a T-shirt to a winter coat.

  - The thicker the layers, the higher the A1c percentage.

Source: American Diabetes Association, *American Diabetes Association Complete Guide to Diabetes: The Ultimate Home Reference from the Diabetes Experts*, 5th ed. (Alexandria, VA: American Diabetes Association, 2011).

My doctor may have adjusted my insulin levels and briefly discussed new insulin therapies or technology. If I wanted to try something new, an educator would visit me. Then a dietitian might drop in with the usual carbohydrate conversation. Nutrition instruction wasn't going to lead to any breakthroughs because I was always approached with the same topic—count carbs, do the math, dose one unit of insulin per fifteen grams of carbs—and that's exactly what I tried to do.

If one could earn a degree in carb counting, I was Dr. Carbohydrate, but if my A1c value wasn't improving, it was assumed that I needed help with Diabetes 101. Problem-solving reminders were fine, but while I continued to try one-way solutions, my body and attitude ventured off-road.

Considering the collection of people who were analyzing me at each visit, it was amazing how much they missed. Complex problems aren't usually solved by continually trying the same approach, but the pathway was marked by narrow standards. The more I felt restricted to the basic diabetes pool, the less stable my mental health became. Whatever they thought worked for everyone wasn't going to cut it with this renegade girl, and bending myself to fit the mold was never going to happen.

Diabetes and Emotions

The human brain is wired to protect us at all times, but it has not evolved to adapt to modern challenges. Our greatest fears today are rooted in emotions, and the fear of being judged is fueled by first impressions. Not only are we visible to the outside world now more than ever, but we are hypercritical of ourselves. Our sense of self-worth is on the line with the pressure we put on ourselves to please others and be accepted.

Burnout is common, and the daily grind of diabetes can certainly put the cherry on top. The best course of action is to acknowledge when overwhelming feelings strike and try to understand where they're coming from. Burnout is tied to how we perceive challenges in life. We may think that ignoring our feelings is a method of fighting back, but that only bottles up tension. The feeling may always be looming if we don't identify what is affecting our attitude and do something to help ourselves.

I have met many overachieving young people with T1D who push themselves to the limit. The combination of a straight-A student and multisport athlete who also plays a musical instrument and volunteers on the weekends is a recipe for perfectionism. Although these young people are focused and disciplined, monitoring blood sugar is sometimes overlooked among the plethora of commitments that distract them from the one thing that isn't always predictable.

Diabetes is unlike a multiple-choice test, or reading music, or becoming a well-trained athlete. Every day can be different, burdensome, and unmeasurable. These are challenging characteristics to accept for someone who excels at calculable things, and frustration can make space for feelings of failure. This is an opportunity to lean into healthy habits that awaken positivity, reframing pessimistic thinking.

The person living with diabetes is not at fault for feeling burned out or distressed. When we feel unheard, unfairly labeled, or threatened with complications because of the numbers that we are measured by, it's hard to feel motivated to meet expectations set by doctors. The institutionalized management of diabetes can make us feel like nothing more than a numerical value measured against rigid standards. Standards don't care how much we may be struggling to cope deep down inside; they exist to measure outcomes that clinical practices are judged by. And this has nothing to do with the emotional well-being of the person.

If we feel like our care team is the problem, we can use our voices to create a positive change. Facing our emotions takes confidence, but asking for help shows that we are aware of our pain. When we begin to think differently about our future, others around us will respond.

**What You Can Do to Support Someone
Going through Diabetes Distress**

- Acknowledge challenges without judgment and offer your ear.

- Take it slowly; allow a person feeling distressed to speak and respond at their own pace.

- Avoid sympathizing with negative statements; "Diabetes sucks," "My life is so hard," "I hate taking insulin," and "I should stop eating carbs" are complaints that can prevent progress.

- Encourage independent thinking and problem-solving.

- Ask permission to share your opinion.

- Allow space but check in regularly to ease the burden of loneliness.

- Keep conversations light without discussing a diabetes-related topic out of the blue.

- Treat a person with T1D individually without comparison to others.

3

THE REBELLION BEGINS

Life's lessons come in many forms

DEALING WITH AUTHORITY while going through puberty with type 1 diabetes is like getting pulled over for speeding—something I became quite accustomed to. When the officer appeared at the window, I handed over my documents and put on my best Disney Princess face. What I'd acted out in the doctor's office was now a pattern I repeated on the highway. I resented authority.

Even though I knew I was doing something wrong, I lied about it. Or at least, softened the truth. Eventually, I learned that resisting the truth only makes a muddy situation worse. And expensive. And time consuming. But speeding was my thing, and an addiction that gave me a sense of freedom. The gas pedal suited my fired-up personality from the moment I hit the highway. I was pulled over for speeding no fewer than a dozen times before I graduated from my parents' insurance policy. Acting careless, reckless, and impatient, with a need-for-speed playlist, was how I rebelled.

The police always asked a variation of the same question: "Do you know how fast you were going?"

How I might have responded, depending on the day: "I'm aware that I accelerated, but I had to get around that minivan. They're dangerous!"

Sometimes the officer laughed. Most of the time, they thought I was an idiot with a lead foot driving a stick shift—not an incorrect observation. Minus the addiction, the main reason I continued to drive fast was that my dad didn't know about most of the tickets. Dad's insurance indicated that I was family to a service member, and that saved my butt. Every once in a while, the officer would write a ticket for a lesser penalty—speeding within ten miles per hour over the speed limit instead of the eighteen I was actually over. Less than ten miles per hour over wasn't reported to insurance, and Commander Plunkett didn't find out.

Although I can admit that I was speeding without remorse, I always tried to make the officer laugh because humor and charm matter when you get busted. If that didn't work with the officer, I went to court to try to talk the ticket down and was usually successful.

I was willing to misbehave as long as I could get away with it or receive a very mild punishment. This was the same approach I took with endocrinology appointments.

THE WAITING ROOM became a busier place as I got into my upper teens. When I started driving myself to appointments, I couldn't help but wonder how many of these kids were newly diagnosed and just starting out on their T1D journey. There always seemed to be more of them and less of me as I looked around. Where were the kids my age? I always wondered why it appeared as if diabetes were only for little kids. We were expected to grow up. *Weren't we?*

Going to appointments by myself meant the care team had to speak directly to me and not over my head to my parents anymore, and that made for a quick visit. Before seeing the doctor, sometimes I'd briefly see a diabetes educator or dietitian. As we hurried over the usual information from repeat handouts, I'd hide my disinterest behind a smile and hand over my blood sugar logbook of mostly made-up numbers.

Did they seriously think I wrote everything down? Lying to my doctors was a return on investment that sped up a visit that was already a lose-lose situation. It took no less than three hours round trip to drive twenty-two miles for a fifteen-minute prodding. And that was without speeding! Considering how closely they observed my physiology through blood testing, little concern was shown for my mental state. This is one reason I was able to avoid talking about my emotions. Feelings take a lot of energy and concentration. Coping with emotions was a drain, and I didn't want to share mine with anyone.

I am certain that I was not alone in withholding information; my body language screamed, *I don't want to be here!* The directive never changed: carb count, take your insulin, come back in three months. And that was fine by me. I wasn't ready to speak up for my actions, and it was easier on everyone if I didn't. Wasn't I doing the clinic a favor by being an unmemorable case to close? The goal never changed: "Do what you're told and come back with better blood sugar control."

Yep, got it.

The only reason I showed up to these visits was to keep my prescriptions updated. I could live without seeing the inside of this clinic ever again, but I couldn't live without insulin.

It was just as much my fault that life wasn't easy, but weren't we all the same when we were kids? If authority came knocking, it was easier to run or lie instead of stepping up. With or without T1D, everyone goes through adolescence and tallies up moments of regret they either wish hadn't happened or can't tell their folks about. My actions demonstrated that I was not ready to be held accountable for my diabetes decision-making practices, yet I thought I was holding it together rather well since expectations were always the same. Numbers and medications were priorities at clinic visits, but what affected my blood sugar the most were the feelings I was battling deep inside. Driving fast and playing sports were outlets that shut my mind off but swept my issues under the rug.

Pushing the authority envelope gave me a thrill, but it extended into nutrition practices that were harmful, creating deep-rooted emotional dilemmas that I denied would ever get in my way.

Caffeine

When I was in high school, a Starbucks opened up in the neighboring suburb. For a twelve-mile drive, I could get a Venti mocha Frappuccino with whipped cream, and it was everything I didn't need going down the hatch. *Hello, dopamine, it's Friday, and I'm here for another hit!* I'd sit and pretend to study while my body labored to make do with the sixty-seven grams of fast-acting sugar I was digesting. That's nearly twice as much sugar as the recommended maximum for a woman my size for an entire day.

Let's be honest: most blended coffee drinks are ALL sugar. Twenty-four ounces of whole milk with four pumps of mocha sauce equals high blood sugar. That adds up to as many calories as a solid meal, with nothing of value digested for sustainable use. If I looked at the label—I never looked at the label—I'd feel guilty. And ignorance was bliss. I'd be home for a nutritious dinner in a few hours, where I could make up my nutrients.

Nutritional denial and carbohydrate assumption was my thing. I'd take some insulin while I was slurping my drink and take another dose for dinner when I got home. Every dose for food was a guess. It took multiple doses of insulin until my blood sugar finally stabilized around bedtime. Between the after-school Frappuccino and getting into bed, my blood sugars were unstable for at least six hours. I had been inactive while doing homework after dinner, but 130 milligrams of afternoon caffeine was still working its magic throughout my system.

The 130 milligrams of caffeine in a twenty-four-ounce serving is nothing compared to the buzz of black coffee, but I never thought that caffeine could affect my blood sugar, sleep quality, or hormones. *But it did, big time.*

I finally learned my lesson with the mocha Frap when I was in college.

I had skipped breakfast to get to class on time. Once freed, I peeled out for Starbucks. I needed a sugar fix really bad after thinking on an empty stomach, and desperation determined that checking my blood sugar was too time consuming. Feeling hungry often made me think my blood sugar was low, but in fact, I was sky high. I ordered the Venti, ate the whipped cream off the top, and took a few heavy slurps of syrupy sugar from the bottom of the cup.

Ahhh, replenished, I thought.

But wait—an unusual feeling grumbled from my esophagus, and within ten seconds, I went from pure bliss to projectile vomiting in my driver's seat. Mocha-whipped upchuck stuck to the door frame and the seatbelt, but I was wearing most of it. I opened the car door to wring out my shirt and continued to vomit clear fluid.

Moral of the story: *ignoring high blood sugar and dosing yourself with a Frappuccino instead of insulin is not sexy.*

Now that I'm all grown up, I order a very responsible coffee drink. I like it better than a Frappuccino because feeling like crap isn't a goal of mine anymore, and rebelling doesn't involve hurting myself. Although, when I started to think outside the box about diabetes, I did make one major sacrifice.

I went decaf.

Insanity. *I know!*

Until the evidence of why it was smart to reduce caffeine presented itself.

IT ALL BEGAN when I desperately started drinking coffee at my part-time hospital job while in nutrition school. The homework load was unbelievable, and desperate times called for desperate measures if I was going to pass biochem. Four o'clock to nine o'clock in the evening was usually a great time for steady blood sugars, but I found myself in need of a correction dose halfway through my shift, even though I had not eaten. This was odd and a bit frustrating. *Why do I need insulin right now?*

The hint at what was happening came from a paramedic pal who sent me on a research rampage. I knew him as a reader of all things medical and as having knowledge that filled him with a reservoir of facts—the kind you might randomly remember when the time is right. One evening, I was whimpering about my blood sugar going up when he pointed at my coffee cup and said, "It's the caffeine. Fight-or-flight is messing with you. Look it up!"

And just like that, regular coffee was a thing of the past.

As I read through a range of studies on caffeine, I became particularly interested in how it boosts athletic performance, and I started to wonder, *Where does the energy behind the caffeine come from?*

This question took me down a complicated path of metabolism, hormones, and performance-enhancing mechanisms of actions—a fancy way of saying that every action has a reaction. Drinking caffeine lights all the systems of the body up like a Christmas tree, along with adrenaline, a hormone that blunts the release of glycogen (stored sugar) from muscles during exercise. *This was the key point to understand.*

Glucose is readily available in the blood, and it's also stored in muscles and the liver. When glucose is stored, we change its name to glycogen. Sports-performance research has found that adrenaline preserves glycogen when exercising, which stimulates fat burn and delays fatigue; this is one reason why athletes have been using caffeine for decades.[7] The *mechanisms of action* have been studied hundreds of different ways to find the optimal use of caffeine for performance enhancement, as every athlete wants to find their competitive edge.

Caffeine may delay the use of glycogen during exercise, but it is not the solution for preventing low blood sugar. We must consider the type of exercise, duration, and intensity to prevent hypoglycemia. See the Exercise section for more information.

Learning about athletes and how caffeine delays fatigue was cool and all, but how was I going to filter this heavy load of information down to something I could understand and relate to myself?

Gimme an eight-ounce serving of knowledge, please.

- Caffeine increases alertness, blood pressure, and heart rate, lasting for several hours depending on individual sensitivity; blood sugar elevates in response to a delay in muscles burning glucose.

- Adrenaline is a hormone triggered by caffeine. The *fight-or-flight* response describes a survival mechanism to react suddenly in life-threatening conditions. Adrenaline is released to spare blood sugar, using fat for energy.

1. The risk of sipping on regular coffee, even without eating carbohydrates, is high blood sugar, and
2. a continuous buzz stimulates adrenaline, causing a prolonged rise in blood sugar.

How Does Caffeine Cause So Much Mayhem?
Caffeine is a stimulant that is absorbed within minutes, triggering full-body reactions. Blood pressure and breathing increase, the mind races, and bowels take action, and many of us can't start our

day without it. A person can build up a tolerance to caffeine with persistent intake, as it stays in the body several hours after ingestion.

According to the Food and Drug Administration (FDA), up to four hundred milligrams of caffeine per day is considered safe, but chronically elevated adrenaline is not okay. Sipping on a bottomless cup of coffee or pounding energy drinks to stay awake can lead to a crash of jitters and insomnia. If this becomes routine, it's an addiction. If specialty coffee drinks are chosen as meal replacements, nutrition will be lacking, and this leads to feeling tired and having little energy. I recommend avoiding this cycle.

The combination of a caffeine buzz, sugar high, and yo-yo blood sugars instead of quality nutrition is a hard pattern to break and stresses the body. Pushing through normal daily activities on poor sleep quality while running on calories from sugar on a routine basis can take a toll on hormones, which prefer not to work overtime.

The evidence leads us to believe that caffeine also spikes insulin levels.

Researchers have been on to the caffeine-and-blood-sugar relationship since a study conducted in 1967 confirmed that blood glucose increases after consuming caffeine. Several studies in the first decade of the 2000s reported the same results. At rest, caffeine lowers insulin sensitivity and impairs the ability of muscles to use glucose in people without diabetes. A study in 2002 found a 25 percent reduction in insulin sensitivity! This would translate to a significant rise in insulin needs for people with diabetes.[8]

Beat the Buzz

To put this into perspective, 95 milligrams per 8 ounces of coffee is considered average, 8 ounces of blonde roast is 180 milligrams, and a cup of decaf is less than 5 milligrams of caffeine. If you're a daily caffeine drinker and you've noticed that it's having an effect on you, scale back slowly.

I love coffee, and some days I need the hard stuff, but it's usually in the form of half-caff: equal parts regular coffee mixed with decaf. I'm sensitive to caffeine, and I notice how it changes my physiology right away because I've drastically decreased from the amount I used to drink. Breakfast is much easier for dosing insulin after eliminating an unpredictable variable like caffeine. I've discovered half-caff to be my threshold, and the result is blood sugar levels more often in range throughout the morning. If I notice the feeling of jitters, my first thought is that I went over my threshold and I'll need to be self-aware of my blood sugars fluctuating over the next few hours.

If you're thinking, *No way am I giving up my strong cuppa joe,* I recommend having it with a meal, not alone. Absorbing complex carbohydrates with any beverage that raises blood sugar and dosing accurately is best practice for minimizing variables like caffeine.

Booze

I may not have wanted to understand the effects of caffeine in high school, but another substance I understood even less was alcohol.

I had a few friends who partied in high school, but it wasn't my thing. Drinking to get sick on purpose was the last thing I was interested in, and I didn't want to find out what would happen if I came home wasted. I wasn't interested in testing limits with substances, but eventually I needed to understand what a drink would do to my blood sugar. By my junior year, I was preparing to move to Florida, so naturally, I'd have to try something with an umbrella and sliced fruit on the rim.

I'd heard stories of freshmen in college with T1D who blacked out after a night of binge drinking and never woke up. Commander Plunkett had already made it very clear that I had a better head on my shoulders than that, but I needed to know if there was more to alcohol than just overconsumption.

KNOW THE THREE Bs: Bread before Booze and don't Black out.

Society challenges itself digestively as a social rite of passage, and we've all done it to some extent. However, the concern about diabetes and alcohol is rather serious. A night of heavy drinking is almost guaranteed to end in rock-bottom-low blood sugar unless a well-timed, balanced meal is eaten. This means we must eat before drinking and absolutely under no circumstances lose consciousness. Alcohol impairs judgment for all, but with T1D, it impairs our ability to respond to low blood sugar. A lack of carbohydrates and a flood of alcohol is the perfect storm for a severe low. If a person passes out while blood sugars are trending down at a rapid rate, the chances of not waking up to treat the low are dangerously high.

Another B is for *buddy*. Drinking pals (especially the designated driver) and a roommate should know the signs of acting unusual due to low blood sugar. Partying is inevitable, but acting uncontrollable should not be. Testing our limits is how we learn, but the best course of action is to firmly establish a few agreements for safety. The eye in the sky via a CGM (continuous glucose monitoring) share app is handy, but I recommend parental boundaries regarding this. College students are adults, and it would be wise to negotiate *when* parents or anyone that can see virtual glucose trends can intervene.

Golden rule: go slow.

Alcohol impairs judgment and rational thinking, and it's a depressant that can affect people in different ways. Avoid trying to keep up with someone who challenges you to drink. Other people are not responsible for the consequences that your body suffers from alcohol poisoning. Best-case scenario—the following day is spent clocking quality time with the toilet and deep breathing in any room that isn't spinning. Being sick and hungover as a result of a night partying beyond being able to remember isn't worth the physical sacrifice. And let's be honest—if you've seen reality TV, you know it's not that cool to get booze-blasted beyond comprehension.

Word to the wise: always look out for yourself and be aware. Being impaired isn't something to aspire to, it's something people get away with until their actions catch up with them.

Real talk: You're planning to sacrifice yourself to the alcohol gods for a particular occasion. What do you do?

1. Carbohydrates have never been more important than in this situation. Eat to slow down alcohol absorption and to prevent an unsuspected low; eat balanced during the day and before going out. Be sure to have access to food and water while drinking and after.
2. If blood sugar appears to be elevated for too long, resist the urge to overadminister insulin while you're drinking. Remember, a correction dose stays in the system for up to three hours. If you have insulin on board and fall asleep without eating enough, a low is highly likely to occur.
3. Heat intensifies the effect of alcohol and also speeds up the rate of insulin absorption! Be aware of alcohol and fast-acting insulin working together—e.g., drinking in a hot tub or while sunbathing.
4. Water, water, water. Stay hydrated while you drink, and replenish well the next day.

I also recommend asking yourself if it's worth it. I can speak with experience on this subject, and I remember exactly how many times I tested my boozy threshold. Those nights will never leave me. No matter how many drinks I'm offered, I know my limit with alcohol, and it will not be pushed. Lapses in memory and losing an entire day because of a hangover are not sexy, nor are they healthy. And as for being out with friends who drink like there's no tomorrow, my advice is to be the responsible one to ensure that there *will* be a tomorrow for you.

Just like a good meal, choose wisely and savor the flavor. There is no glory in waking up in a strange place, sleeping in a jail cell, or, heaven forbid, not waking up at all.

4

SHIPWRECKED ON
DIABETES ISLAND

No matter how far you travel, you cannot run from yourself

THREE WEEKS AFTER graduating high school, I made the very grown-up decision to leave home and venture into the wild. I moved into my own apartment in Florida, started college full-time, and worked at a restaurant with an ocean view. I was never more than ten minutes from the beach, feeling warm ocean breezes everywhere I went.

It was paradise.

Seven Minnesota winters I lived through, seven years of beach time it would take to thaw out.

My plan was to make a life on the seashore, and I was determined to see it through, but taking care of my diabetes wasn't exactly on the self-improvement radar. I knew nothing about the effects of caffeine or alcohol yet. Everything was an uneducated experiment from here. Sun worshipping 1,500 miles away from the kid clinic of the past, I felt a nagging responsibility to find an adult endocrinologist, but it was definitely not an urgent priority. I was a working student, exploring my new coastal neighborhood, and mingling with handsome coast guards. You know, the important things. And there was no reason to rush. I had enough diabetes supplies stocked up to get through at least a year. I was finally free of the expectation to be seen by a doctor every three months, and it was liberating. *Turning eighteen rules!* I had the rest of my life to figure out diabetes, and inviting another doctor into my life could wait. For now, I was going to revel in rebellion and rock out with my tan lines out.

It didn't take long for my naive independence to clash with a lack of maturity. I was darn responsible for my age, but I wasn't in the best control of my emotions. My temper was maxed out, as evidenced by the dozen-plus speeding tickets I had deserved, along with routine verbal outbursts and door slamming. The neighbors heard numerous volatile phone calls about prescriptions, homework, and bills, and random outbursts with discarded boyfriends. They occasionally checked in, knowing that I lived alone, and I suppose they wanted to confirm that the horrible sounds were not evidence of an exorcism. Nope, just a young adult trying to navigate grown-up stuff and wondering why life wasn't easier in such a beautiful place. In hindsight, the continuous roller coaster of fluctuating blood sugars had a lot to do with my reactive personality.

Being present in my environment was the healthy outlet for my internal frustrations. Going to the beach, rollerblading in the park, or driving the coastline made up for bad days. Unhealthy outlets included lots of chocolate and people watching with a sugar-loaded specialty coffee drink in hand. And because of it, I'd spend the rest of the day trying to lower my blood sugar. There were no consequences to my self-destructive behaviors. That's the advantage of being a loner. Avoiding responsibilities and numbing my thoughts was a delay tactic that set me back more and more each day, but I felt like I was solving problems on my own.

My choices were causing harm, but I thought I was normalizing the duties of diabetes by acting like nothing bad could happen. *Look, world, I can eat chocolate and still keep my eyesight intact and my toes attached.* I didn't have the knowledge I needed to command my health, and I took risks to spite the direction I historically had been given. My daily constant was inconsistency, and the only reason I would ever see blood sugar in healthy range was because of dumb luck.

It seemed to take a lot of effort to have a mediocre day, and to my understanding, everything I wanted to eat was bad for me. *And the more I told myself it was bad, the more I wanted it.*

My solution for living with diabetes was to be an opposing force rather than compromise at a midpoint.

After a year without appointments, my supplies were dwindling and I needed updated prescriptions to get affordable insulin. The fact that I needed the equivalent of a permission slip for medications that I would otherwise die without made me very angry. Shouldn't supplies for incurable diseases be the lowest-hanging fruit? Maybe somewhere over the rainbow. But in the United States, medical insurance sets the mode and cadence at which diabetes supplies are distributed. And it sucks. Even if you're healthy and have insurance, living with diabetes is still expensive.

I had no choice but to obey to stay alive, and there was no time to waste. Running out of insulin was a frightening thought, followed by, *Buck up, kid. You're in charge of you now.*

I was committed to taking grown-up measures, so I found a doctor who I was willing to start fresh with. However, surviving alone with diabetes was a burden beginning to engulf me. The feeling that rested heavy on my shoulders was loneliness.

There was no graduation ceremony from the colorful pediatric facility or welcome transition into the barren cavity that is an adult clinic. Other than washed-out pictures of boats and beaches on the walls, my new endocrinology office was a drab whitewash that smelled like old magazines and alcohol wipes. I had stranded myself on an imaginary island where almost-adults with T1D go to sink or swim. I was as good as marooned on Diabetes Island.

DIABETES ISLAND WAS established long before I arrived. The inhabitants with badges were set in their ways and not easily impressed, nor were they accepting of challengers. I was exposed, but ignored. Examined, but overlooked. Listened to, but not heard. The confusion of it all lashed out from under the shelter of my parents as an ex-pediatric patient. I may have just entered the world of adulting with diabetes, but I was hoping to wade into the shallow end before diving in headfirst. Shivers of isolation and vulnerability shot down from head to toe with one lightning bolt of a thought: *Holy shit. I'm officially dealing with diabetes on my own. WILSON, where are you?!*

On the Island, my new doctor never smiled. I was lucky to get eye contact before the tone of disappointment filled the room. Body language included a lot of head-shaking statements: "Your control is not good," "Your thyroid is going to go," "You should not eat that." But I kept showing up to appointments like a glutton for punishment. I was prescribed an insulin pump and took a few classes to learn how to use it safely. The words *basal* and *bolus* entered my vocabulary to describe the difference between insulin constantly trickling from the pump and the larger dose I needed specifically for meals. Using the pump instead of taking insulin injections was cool at first, but my A1c reached double digits. I gained more weight, I felt exhausted, and my long hair was disintegrating. I was screaming for help on the inside, but "Dr. Frost" had a way of neutralizing emotions inside the sterilized icebox of an interrogation.

I told myself that I didn't need coddling because I was adulting, but a pleasant disposition shouldn't be exclusive to kids. She was as cold as January in the frozen northland and brought the chill of winter into the exam room. As I waited in uncomfortable silence, the click of heels in the hallway signaled the walls to turn to ice.

Anyone that may have known me on a brighter day would've thought I was really, really sad.

I wasn't offering up my feelings, but if the blood work doesn't lie, it shouldn't have taken much to notice how bad off I was. As a new pumper, I had to check in every three months with Dr. Frost and found myself right back where I left off, with frequent visits going nowhere. The only difference was the three hundred units of insulin strapped to my hip for all to see.

The pump wasn't making me healthier, smarter, or more confident, as the last drop of positive energy I was clinging to evaporated. Despite the way I looked and felt, my mediocre attempt at diabetes management got a passing grade from within the clinic because I had demonstrated pump proficiency. I tested my blood sugar and knew how to change pump settings, and that was good enough. I tried to drop hints that I didn't like the pump, but I usually left appointments feeling more confused than I had been to begin with.

"Hey, Doc, I woke up covered in blood and realized the insertion came out during the night. I placed a new pump site, but my blood sugar was high the entire next day and I felt terrible."

"Mm-hmm, sounds like you know what to do, and be sure to eat less carbs. Do you need updated prescriptions, Lauren?"

"Huh?"

I guess I should expect a shitty day after bleeding from my stomach all night.

"No, I'm good."

The bar was set about an inch higher than rock bottom, so I carried on with the same habits and I wasn't dead yet—quite the measurable goal, but I wanted better for myself, and I couldn't continue feeling beyond frustrated. *Why couldn't I get this blood sugar thing under control?!*

Depression

The prevalence rates of depression can be up to three times higher in patients with T1D.[9] Depression can worsen disease, while the daily responsibility of diabetes can lead to feelings of depression, a pattern that encircles the mental health of a person with diabetes. Chronic stress, poor sleep, and persistent worrying can cause hormones to become overactive. This may lead to cravings and

Ten Questions to Ask Yourself if You Suspect Depression Is Disrupting Your Life

To create resolutions, circle each question you are experiencing and assign a number to indicate how strongly you feel about it: 1 is the lowest effect; 5 is the highest effect. The questions with the highest effects are priorities to take immediate care with.

- Am I feeling down?

- Has my appetite changed?

- Am I sleeping a lot or very little?

- Is my energy low?

- Do I feel agitated or angry?

- Am I having a hard time concentrating or making decisions?

- Do I feel helpless or guilty?

- Are my thoughts toward myself negative?

- Have I stopped having fun?

- Do I have thoughts of hurting myself?

For immediate help coping, visit Crisistextline.org or text HOME to 741741.

This exercise is a process in self-awareness that provides a starting point for self-care that may branch into conversations about mental health. Talk to someone you trust about your feelings. Before speaking with a friend or professional, it may help to write down what you want to say, including one to three things you need that would help you heal.

overeating to soothe the pain. When depression and stress are unrelenting, unhealthy habits are easy to fall on.

Feeling depressed does not mean you are broken or less than. Examine your thoughts, write them down, tell someone when you're ready, and chin up to finding solutions. You are brave and you can face this.

Positive self-talk is a practice that includes visualization and self-care as methods of coaching yourself. The inner coach, as opposed to the inner critic, builds self-awareness and strengthens our ability to adapt to difficult experiences. Come as they may, when we are our best coach, tough days sail by with the wind as we stand firm.

Occasional sadness triggered by certain events can escalate into depression. I could admit that I felt sad, and that my eating habits were a major source of my sour mood, lack of energy, and poor body image. I could no longer go at this alone, and once I decided to talk about it, it felt like a weight had lifted from my shoulders. The time had finally arrived to get insightful and start taking a serious look at what I was struggling with, because otherwise Dr. Frost could be the end of me.

I of the Hurricane

As insulin pumps became the popular choice in diabetes technology, the flexibility of faster-acting insulin provided the opportunity to improve blood sugar time in range. This led to expectations for lower A1c, and I was intrigued. If it was possible to improve blood sugar on the pump, I was willing to try, but that would require a change.

Using the pump and managing insulin was clearly a priority, but food was the bane of my existence. I knew how seriously I was supposed to take nutrition, but the topic of eating was the most sensitive subject. Keeping food records would have been evidence of my failure, and I wasn't ready to see what I was putting in my body written on paper—that would have made my mistakes real. Food records would force me to look myself straight in the eyes and admit that I was letting diabetes own me. The truth is, I didn't know where to start.

My appetite was either nonexistent or full throttle like I'd never been fed. A standard day was cereal and milk in the morning, a peanut butter sandwich in the afternoon, junk in between meals to soothe my sweet tooth, and a late dinner. I often spent my shift at the restaurant guzzling regular soda as the rush of customers dropped my blood sugar like a rock. I didn't have a plan for preventing lows, so I'd disconnect my pump, completely stopping the flow of insulin. Once insulin is in, you can't take it out, so I figured it was better to cut off my supply for a little while.

Hours later when I reconnected the line, I battled highs that seemed to never come down. The overflow of regular soda plus high blood sugar made me feel sick to my stomach, so I'd go to bed without eating, yet stuffed with liquid sugar.

I was acutely aware that I could have better control, but life was starting to interfere with my better judgment. Variables like staying up late, going out with friends, eating whatever I wanted, and stress were taking a toll on my body. Making the mistake of dosing myself for meals with too much insulin, or too little, had a domino effect that dropped my energy level. Every proactive decision was a shot in the foot that I had either overestimated or underestimated.

Taking fast-acting insulin at the right time seemed impossible with my schedule and unpredictable chemistry. The only thing I could count on happening was force-feeding myself to compensate for the insulin that would continue to absorb for the next several hours. I was stuck in an energy-sucking cycle of insulin imbalance and calorie overload. I called it "chasing my tail," which I did every day, all day.

The medical term for it is *overinsulinization*, followed by overtreating hypoglycemia, followed by guilt and disappointment.

The blood sugar roller coaster was draining the life from me, but I didn't know any other way to manage. Every day was like living in the eye of a hurricane, life swirling around me, waiting for it to get worse. Sure, I could've been more disciplined, but did it really matter what I ate if diabetes wasn't going anywhere?

This was a storm that had no end in sight. I was willing to keep working at it, but I was drowning.

Work and school began to lose their luster, as plans for the future were caving, and I was too angry to recognize paradise anymore. Back at the clinic, Diabetes Island was determined to crack me like a seashell, but I was still hanging on and trying to navigate my way through the transition to becoming an adult. No matter how frosty my doctor was, if I could weather this, it would be smooth sailing from here on out. *It had to be!*

And then came the cascade of epic meltdowns.

The buttons stopped working on my first pump.

A few months later, the replacement malfunctioned during a flight to Paris.

Suddenly realizing that my pump died was a next-level nightmare and yet another adventure seemingly set up by the Island to test my capacity to put up with an accumulating pile of you-know-what. I had to drop everything, make the necessary calls, and wait it out. My doctor gave me a crash course on switching over to insulin injections while waiting for a new pump to arrive.

I didn't mind going back to injections, but I needed a different kind of insulin and immediate change of protocol to avoid putting myself in a worse situation than I was already in.

Events like this were destroying me, piece by piece, and I was beginning to wonder what I was working so hard for. I wasn't going to call home crying and worry my parents more than they already were. Nor could they solve my problems any faster than I could. I got myself into this; I had to get myself out. However, a silver lining emerged while navigating through Hurricane Diabetes. Spearheading the range of adventures in supplies taught me how to speak healthcare fluently. I learned all about insulin, pumps, and insurance, but I still wasn't getting anywhere with my personal health.

My rebellious habits with food were peaking with increasing portions of junk food to soothe my emotions. I treated Hershey's Kisses and Cheerios like they were food groups, and I accidentally lit my oven on fire trying to cook onion rings. Lean Cuisine meals never satisfied my appetite, and some days a coffee-loaded milkshake and Diet Coke were my only form of nourishment.

I never looked forward to meeting with Dr. Frost, but this time I asked for help with my nutrition. If there was anything I didn't learn as a kid, it was how to avoid gaining weight, since that's all I did from the moment I was diagnosed. I had an A+ in chubby anger, and that was about it. I was so ashamed of my body for all the effort it took to keep myself alive. Feeling down and out with fear and shame is what caused me to step back from trying anything new, isolate, and wall myself in.

I wanted to lower my A1c because I wanted to shove it in Frost's face. She didn't believe in me, and I was sick of feeling like a diabetes dropout. My attitude was terrible, and even if I lowered my A1c, it would take a miracle for Frost to thaw out with an improved bedside manner.

I had to want to be healthy for myself.

It was time to go on a soul-searching expedition to discover who I wanted to be and find the person living in the shadow of diabetes.

5

FEEDING THE DISEASE

Food was the problem and the solution

ON THE INDEPENDENT road to self-discovery, I was beginning to realize there were two things I needed to lift my spirit: *personalized education and a healthy example of life with diabetes.*

I felt defeated by the chore that eating had become, and though my world revolved around food, I didn't know how to apply what I knew about nutrition to change my lifestyle.

Blood sugar and nutrition must be on the same wavelength for health to flourish, starting with determining knowledge gaps and separating food facts from fiction. Taking inventory of what I thought I knew left me with more questions than answers:

Whole foods—*what's that mean?*

What was that special thing about fiber? *Something about magical fruit . . .*

If I only eat one meal a day, does it matter what it is? *In other words, can I just eat cake?*

Diet soda is a substitute for water, right? *Clueless.*

I'd had dozens of one-on-one experiences with dietitians and diabetes educators by the time I reached Diabetes Island. These visits were a source of deeply rooted and painful memories that I associated with "food rules" and diabetes education. The direction I was given made sense to the provider, but to me, the glove didn't fit. Routinely, I found myself learning from the uninspired and disengaged, agenda-driven employee who clocked out of diabetes at the end of the day. I left each appointment with the same humdrum nutrition handout and without an ounce of motivation.

Taking insulin with meals may as well have been a shot in the dark. My brain would tell me to use a measuring cup for portion control, while my appetite raged to eat more. Try as I might to rationalize my decisions, food was the enemy. Eating wasn't about enjoyment or energy, but rather a survival tool that delivered unrelenting punishment. Historically, the meal plan I was told to follow was aligned with the government-standardized United States Department of Agriculture (USDA) food pyramid. The daily recommended servings suggested that I should eat set portions of the five food groups. I was given a plan to eat three meals and snacks daily with specific serving amounts. Although I appreciate that a nutrition strategy would have helped me, the rules and expectations were set to a nonnegotiable, one-size-fits-all standard, lacking in flexibility. Sounds easy, but the plan had flaws.

The first huge problem: The number of daily servings recommended by dietitians was more than what I needed to maintain a healthy body weight at my age, and eating too many calories leads to weight gain.

The second huge problem: The expectation to be absolutely precise in portions and carb count with every single meal left little wiggle room. And let's be honest, using measuring cups or a scale every single time is not realistic.

Everything I put in my mouth was supposed to be measured, counted, and portioned. Some foods were called "free" when they contained less than five grams of carbohydrates per serving, while other carbs had to be restricted to a certain amount per meal.

My mind was crawling with *why*s, and the pathway of blood sugar control was as foggy as ever. Being told to restrict carbohydrates without understanding why made me feel worse, and I wasn't aware of any other solution. It was like being trapped on a sinking raft that, while trying to repair the puncture, I unintentionally put more holes in. There was always an event, a mistake, a "whoops, shouldn't have eaten that" moment in my day.

Specific nutrition to support my activity level was never discussed. However, the conversation steered toward damage control as a result of exercise, which presented as evidence for how often I failed at balancing physical activity, nutrition, and insulin. Attempting to control the variables was like juggling while jumping on a trampoline, and it was taking a toll on my body. My legs always hurt when I ran, my energy level was inconsistent, I lacked focus, and anger fueled my performance. My blood sugar records and elevated A1c determined that I was a "poorly controlled" patient—also known as the diabetes version of a catch-22.

If eating healthy and exercising were the best habits for me, *why weren't they working?*

If the "diabetic diet" was so serious, how come results varied, and why didn't it come with a warning label about how I'd feel about myself? There had to be somebody out there who understood what I was going through, but I didn't know a single person with T1D.

So here I was, preparing to meet the dietitian with the hope that this would finally change the sense of failure I felt around food, exercise, and my body.

Over the years, a constant cause of frustration was the focus on "feeding the disease" as diabetes became my identity. I felt viewed as a diabetic first and a human being second.

There is a fine line between maintaining healthy blood sugar levels and developing an unhealthy relationship with food due to an obsession with control. Guilt by association is common: the feeling that if a certain food causes blood sugar to fluctuate that it is "bad" or "harmful" to eat. In turn, the "bad" foods can become an obsession. And this is where I landed in rebellion against the diabetes food rules. Throwing my hands up in angry surrender and numbing out while mindlessly eating junk that I knew would do more harm than good.

Misery loves company, and that's what snacks were for.

Mirror Image

Just when I thought I was ready to pull up to the table of new beginnings, a defining event swooped in and knocked the chair out from underneath me. I was shaken, and it was the worst of the best disasters that had to happen to wake me up.

I had limited trust in all those with nutrition credentials. In fact, *trust* is a generous word. Registered dietitians exemplified the standing order for my limited confidence and poor body image. In honesty, I was holding on to deep, dark, unforgiving contempt. Attempting to rise above history, I put on my big-girl vulnerability jacket and prepared to tell all for future's sake. The desire to get healthy was brewing in my heart, and I was agreeable to meeting a dietitian who Dr. Frost recommended because it was the last option. If I wasn't prepared to start talking about the pain inside, no one else would.

I checked into a silent and dimly lit hospital lobby on a late afternoon. Judging by the echoing slap of my flip-flops, I was alone. So there was no mistaking the intent of a young blond woman wearing a hospital badge walking straight toward me. She was the dietitian.

The clear coil caught my eye as I spotted an insulin pump on her hip. *Ah-ha, she gets it!*

Yet I was facing a moral dilemma. She introduced herself quietly and softly shook my hand, and I followed her toward a seating area. As we ascended a small staircase, my first impression of her lay heavy on my chest. I saw thinning hair, a blemished complexion, and obvious discomfort in the way she pulled at the clothes that clung to her body. I intuitively understood her without having met her before. She was bubbly and kind, yet shy, and she avoided eye contact. It was as if she read my mind about irony taking shape and sitting at the table with us.

I wanted to ignore what I was thinking, but there was no denying that I was facing a slightly older but significantly heavier version of myself with similar insecurities. My face turned bright red in a fluster, and my heart was in my throat. I wanted to flee.

Diabetes Island was testing me once again. Was my future already determined? Should I find comfort in relating to someone who knows how hard diabetes is and forget about finding solutions? Is it a fantasy to think that a healthy example of someone living with diabetes exists?

I felt hopeless and started to sink into my dark side. My interpretation of the contrast sitting before me was that a nutrition professional with T1D did not appear to be living a healthy life, and she was supposed to have all the answers. I was crushed and demoralized at the prospect of my mirror image, and I was guilty of sizing her up, but the inspiring example I was looking for was not supposed to look like me.

I was being judgmental, but I needed a healthy person to look up to, and she was my last hope. I was finally ready to talk about the ugly personal stuff, but not like this. I had barely skimmed the surface when I told her I wanted to be a healthier size, and I listened to her suggestions, but the bar of expectations was dropping by the second. The references, handouts, and carb-restricting undertones were exactly the same as I'd heard before. I felt like I was melting alive as I began warping into the past, realizing that my greatest fear was true: *Even a dietitian living with diabetes doesn't have the answers.*

Fifteen minutes later, the meeting awkwardly ended and channeled into a reckless drive home. It's a miracle that I didn't get another speeding ticket after I peeled out of the hospital in a hysterical rage. The speeding tantrum made evident my complete loss of faith in the people who had literally been telling me how to stay alive since I was eleven years old. It was a hopeless attempt to believe this visit would be anything different.

I forgot why I was in Florida to begin with, and all I wanted to do was disappear, or turn north. I was only twenty-two hours from a place where I could put my head on my mom's lap and cry. But even she wouldn't have known what to do with this puddle of sadness I'd become. I was absolutely finished. Burnt to a crisp. Beyond consoling. My hemoglobin A1c was in the double digits, the insulin pump was making life harder by the day, and I still didn't know how to eat without making everything worse.

Shipwrecked. Alone. Defeated. Useless.

Diabetes Island was taking no prisoners, and I was up Sugar Creek without a paddle.

An Exercise in Emotional Eating

Keep a three-day food record to observe your habits. This can be scary, but it is an honest way to take responsibility for your food choices privately. If you're struggling to face your food records, it may be time to reach out for help. To build confidence in facing your barriers, I recommend four methods to try individually or in sequence:

- Guided meditation

- Talk therapy

- Low-impact exercise in a nature setting

- One-on-one education with a dietitian

Keep your food log super simple. Each day, list the time, what you ate, and how it made you feel. Words like *bored, starving, stressed,* or *fulfilled after eating* are valuable observations. This record will become a roadmap to your emotions and food choices. Seeing it for yourself can help you make better decisions that are less emotionally driven, while the four methods can help you gain insight on healthy practices specific to your needs.

Breakthrough

My outlook on diabetes became darker by the second as I sat on the floor of my apartment in a spiral of negative thoughts, as the demons of body hatred whispered into my ear. I bawled over my thinning hair, the shape of my body, and the work it took to keep this thing alive.

Who was I if not tied to the value that my glucose monitor displayed? I could wake up one morning feeling inspired with a blood sugar of 100, and feeling worthless the next morning at 399. Limiting myself was a natural defense when I could blame diabetes for crushing every dream I had of traveling Europe and becoming a creative entrepreneur. I once envisioned island-hopping to Balearic beats and filling up on inspiration from the historical landscape. But without loving myself enough to try, I attracted the wrong people and accepted a quality of life that wasn't up to my standards.

Florida was supposed to become my forever home, and there was so much I loved about it. I had visions of living by the beach in a yellow cottage with a big goofy dog, a flower garden, and a closet full of bohemian sundresses. Yet paradise faded into nonexistence as darkness took over the light.

My dreams changed shape like clouds in the wind. One moment I could remember what I wanted, but then it morphed into something I could no longer recognize when I tested my blood sugar.

I was flailing at rock bottom, drowning in self-pity, and pondering the option to drive my pathetic bones north to Minnesota. If I had ruby slippers, I was clicking my heels together hard enough to split them open.

Why am I so miserable? I hate everything. No one gets it. I'm alone. Why am I out of chocolate?!

Just when I thought I would spontaneously combust from overthinking, an extraordinary calm came over me. I'd gone cold with tears and had nothing left to purge. My mind emptied in stillness, but a thought broke through as if fingers snapped in front of my eyes. The constant in all this mayhem was me, and I could no longer run away from myself.

I had reached a turning point while the surrender to emptiness created space for a breakthrough. Even though I was consumed with anger and frustration, I could sense the way out. I was standing at a fork in the road, and I'd weighed the options: *give up or wake up.*

With nothing to look forward to and no plan for the future, I became a blank slate and saw things clearly. I may have been broken, but I refused to stay that way. Nor would I continue to walk the same path. I couldn't remember the last time I laughed, and the ridiculousness of how unacceptable that was triggered a reworking. *Wake up and remember who you are, Lauren.*

I was ready to find purpose in this life of disease.

No more food rules and feeling like a failure.

No more being told what to do without understanding why.

No more negative self-talk or allowing the health system to label me unfairly.

Nobody was going to make me feel like I wasn't capable.

I was not going to accept being treated like I would never improve.

Maybe I could change all this—my health, my direction in life, my attitude. Starting with the first thing on the list to change: *Dr. Frost.*

I was getting off this Island on my own two feet with middle fingers pointed to the sky.

Above all, it was time to embrace diabetes like I never had before. *But first, the beach.*

Beachside Baptism

After a storm, driftwood can be found bobbing about the ocean and washed up on the shore. Some pieces of wood are full of character, sparking creativity in beachcombers who give the wood life again as a work of art.

I was embarrassed that I'd ended up like driftwood after all the effort it took to live in paradise. I went to the beach looking for inspiration, but it also felt like a familiar course in another attempt to run away from myself. Only this time, experience had taught me that diabetes would follow.

It took weeks to reflect on the meeting with my mirror-image dietitian and to recover from the memories it triggered. Although I was motivated to turn the corner toward a more positive path, my mind was buzzing with the unknown. I was still standing in the same place: same diabetes, same challenges.

My final assessment was that my life resembled a fire swamp. The palm trees were quite lovely, never mind the rodents of unusual size disguised as guys asking me out and the slimy orcs I worked for. To afford my apartment by the sea, I worked at a busy restaurant famous for gigantic portions of everything—not exactly supportive of my desire to make healthy choices. Eventually, I stopped showing up to that grotesquerie after I learned everything I needed to know about unprofessional management. A person can learn just as much from bad examples as good ones, and I was learning from the best of the worst scumbags in the industry, including those I considered friends.

I was close with several coworkers, who would unwind at my place after shifts. We had a lot of fun together until it was brought to my attention that one of them was stealing my insulin syringes to inject illegal drugs. The person who tipped me off about the conniving thief was the drug dealer himself (also a coworker). He took sympathy knowing that the syringes were mine.

Stone-cold doctors, dirtbag restaurant managers, swindling servers, and sympathetic drug dealers—every day was an experience at *The Lauren Show*!

At the time, it would have been enlightening to know that you attract the energy that you give off. I was aware of the solitary position I had put myself in and that I was a total bummer without an outlet for my pain. I kept diabetes to myself and avoided finding a tribe of my own because I didn't want to talk about my issues.

Uncharacteristically, I got up early one morning and drove to a quiet part of the beach. I laid my towel out and walked across the soft white sand and into the ocean to breathe. Eyes closed and waist deep, sniffing at the warm, salty air to quiet my thoughts. The glistening blue water moved through my fingers as I stood present in my skin, as the beach girl I always wanted to be. I took in the distant horizon, intuitively feeling as though I might never see this place again. My mind began to wander, thinking about the history across the water, to the continent on the other side—maybe that's where I should go next.

Even as I dragged myself through life trying to ignore traumatic memories, I managed to hold on to a sliver of myself underneath the dreadful shame. When I allowed myself to feel present, a little light inside would guide me with brief reminders of what I loved about the world: dreams of traveling to historic sites, watching pelicans dive, and joking with the retired locals; how far I was out from under my parents' roof, where there was always something to chuckle about, a good book to read, and great music. Drifting felt really nice . . .

Then a commotion in the water startled my eyes open.

Two young men about fifty feet to my left were gasping at each other, pointing into the water with looks of sheer panic. Their eyes followed what they were watching as heads swiveled in my direction.

And then I saw it.

A massive black shadow in the shallow water, aimed straight toward me.

Time stood still as I thought, *I've got the sweetest blood out of anyone around here. I'm a goner.*

I looked over at the young men, who undoubtedly thought they were about to witness a massacre, as I stood paralyzed with curiosity more than fear. My instincts told me that this massive black shadow wasn't out for an insulin-deficient morsel. I almost didn't care either way given my complete lack of self-worth. I was ready to donate my body to the nourishment of a water animal since I was a failure at nourishing myself.

This would be my purpose; breakfast for a sea creature.

The dark blue cloud was buoyantly moving closer just below the surface as it slowly started to rise. Flesh was about to crest, so close I could almost touch it. The water suddenly rippled to make way for the fifteen rows of teeth I expected, but instead, long whiskers and a rounded snout rolled to the sky, projecting a forceful shower of ocean spray!

A manatee?! The dark blue death cloud I thought was coming to drag me to Hades was a playful and gigantic frolicking sea cow. I do believe the creature smiled and winked at the sight of my gaping face. Close enough to slap me with a flipper—I'll be gosh darned. *I'm alive!*

Checking to see if my pulse was slowing down, I glanced over my right shoulder at the beach and saw parents pulling their kids away from the water. Yet they were simultaneously realizing that I wasn't being ripped to shreds by a shark, Nessie, or screeching eels. All the while, this gorgeous sea cow was putting on a show: barrel-rolling with flippers surfacing one at a time and spraying water with every turn down the coastline.

It was a manatee's world, and I was happy to be waist deep in it. *Nature is amazing!*

I felt so happy. I lay back to float weightlessly in reflection. Maybe I had just found my tribe; seeing as I had exchanged friends for a sea cow, I was basically mermaid Ariel.

Test strips? I got twenty. But who cares? No big deal. I want moooore.

I continued to float until the worry wheel inside my mind began firing up to reality, but this time something felt different. My manatee friend did something in the transfer of nervous energy that reminded me that I can stand my ground. I wasn't raised to retreat when life gets hard or a little scary, and I could move forward. I knew that I had the qualities to stand up to others if I had to. Yet, why wasn't I standing up for myself?

My emotions had been spinning like a pinwheel. Was the solution really as simple as doing something I enjoyed to penetrate my sadness? All I had to do was take a few big inhales of salt water and briefly fear for my life to receive a powerful sign that would stick with me forever.

Manatees symbolize gentleness, intelligence, and regeneration—three emerging elements that I needed to turn inward to move forward. Focusing on what I failed to accomplish took up more space than it deserved. I needed to care about myself and become an expert of my own body, beginning with a sparkly new attitude.

From the dreadful feelings of defeat, shame, and anger blossomed the unfamiliar feeling of self-reliance. Not only was I going to embrace diabetes, but I would no longer accept the sufferable tone of my diagnosis, or that I should live in fear of complications. What I needed was to become the owner and primary decision maker of my treatment. I was going to demolish the existing structure and run this operation myself.

Diabetes is my disease, and I'm taking agency over my future.

The day of the manatee became a lesson in gratitude and inner dialogue. I was cruel to myself and I knew it, which was the first thing that needed to stop. But I had to start changing my habits on the outside in order to mend what was broken on the inside. This is when I began to take the first steps toward learning how to heal and determining my own experiences in life.

6

THE CORNERSTONES

Blood sugar, nutrition, exercise, and insulin

I WAS FEROCIOUSLY QUICK to erupt for various reasons that funneled into frustration. Going through the same process for years without getting better results was a daily trigger. Making decisions about the cornerstones of diabetes—*blood sugar, nutrition, exercise,* and *insulin adjustments*—requires advanced skills, and I didn't have them. The pressure was on to start making changes, but I was in trouble and I had catching up to do.

Results of a study that examined how young adults aged eighteen to twenty-nine years feel about living with diabetes were similar to my experience. Participants expressed having the need for a personalized experience and difficulty juggling life's priorities with diabetes management that is often unheard in adult care. Balancing the irregular schedule of college life with academic and social obligation presents a new source of distress. Adapting to a new environment and community of people who may not understand life with diabetes adds to the pressure to fit in. For those entering the workforce, diabetes creates a dilemma between job demands and time management. While fear of low blood sugars in the middle of a busy day persists in all age groups, a consistent trend among career-oriented people is challenges with work-life balance as diabetes becomes a lower priority, followed by feeling guilty if blood sugar control declines.[10]

Like myself, young adults often leave the pediatric clinic without establishing a new doctor to transition to. Once they arrive in the adult clinic, a lack of communication between pediatric and adult care further disconnects the transition and creates a barrier for individualized education. Emerging adults with T1D often need behavior and lifestyle support that clinics lack the resources to provide. Nor do clinics have the staff to accommodate the volume of patient requests. Many diabetes-education specialists and adult endocrinologists agree that this age group is time consuming and poorly prepared for self-care, yet few clinics provide programs that help new patients navigate the transition.[11]

Clinics simply can't provide what they don't have. An inefficient clinical model that lacks time and resources forces patients to adapt to the system regardless of their personal needs. This method fails patients as they blend into the mounting workload of practitioners while their health goals remain stagnant.

A study in Australia presented experiences of people between the ages of eighteen and thirty-five living with T1D. Many participants felt they learned by piecemeal education with gaps in knowledge, lacked access to registered dietitians, and had very little access to psychologists. The majority wanted education specialists to acknowledge the difference between self-management theory and the *real-life* experience of living with type 1 diabetes. Ninety-six percent of participants reported accessing resources about diabetes education independent of their healthcare team, including one of the major sources of frustration that is near and dear to my heart: locating information about healthy blood sugars during exercise.[12]

Individually, we all handle diabetes differently, and we can learn a lot from the evidence. Our life experiences as kids going into adult care provides a full-spectrum perspective that is valuable for clinicians to understand. Clarify your expectations by talking with your healthcare team about what you want to accomplish with their help. And if they are not equipped to support you, there are other options for getting the care you deserve.

Blood Sugar and Weight Gain

Diabetes challenges the head, heart, and physical body. Psychological distress, fear of lows, and disordered habits with food are quite common.

I was walking a fine line, with warning signs that could have amplified into harmful behaviors at any moment. Many of my thoughts were unhealthy, but I never ignored my blood sugar, and that is where my frustrations grew seismically—no matter what I did, diabetes was an uphill battle. Fortunately, I was grounded enough to know when to check my thoughts before manipulating insulin levels. I didn't like the feeling of hyperglycemia, and I wasn't prepared to suffer just to lose weight.

The fear of lows and weight gain as a result of taking insulin is widespread. Sometimes this can lead to insulin restriction and harmful practices that increase the risk of complications. Research conducted over a span of eleven years with 234 women living with T1D found that 30 percent reported restricting insulin.[13] These women also had higher body weight and elevated A1c levels despite taking less insulin than they knew they should. This study also found that women who restricted insulin had a mean age of only forty-five years. In fact, 26 of the 234 women passed away before the study could conclude.

Restricting insulin is not the answer for weight loss. In theory, starving cells of glucose forces body fat to be used for energy, but only in exchange for very high blood sugar levels, stressed organs, brain fog, and a shorter life span.

Food is the solution to hypoglycemia, and when survival depends on eating fast-acting carbohydrates as soon as possible, weight gain can be even more disheartening. Bouncing from low to high and back again confuses metabolism as messages are lost in translation. Our appetite can become difficult to interpret once we've trained ourselves to eat without feeling hungry. *Overinsulinization* happens when we have to take extra insulin due to overeating.

In my experience, not only did I have to overeat if I took too much insulin, but I also felt hungry when I could sense that my blood sugar was falling from a high level. The less balanced my insulin was, and the more erratic my blood sugar, the more I wanted to eat. My appetite was unpredictable, and I wasn't skilled enough to balance the cornerstones strategically.

Research from 2015 examined a collection of studies that looked at the prevalence of eating disorders in adolescents with T1D. Generally, risk increases with age; up to 40 percent of young adult females are affected by disordered eating habits.[14] Weight preoccupation, perfectionism, trouble self-regulating, and self-blame are personality characteristics that frequently align within T1D territory. "Bad" foods might be craved and binged in rebellion, and episodes of low blood sugar can lead to overeating foods that may otherwise be restricted, sparking feelings of guilt, followed by further restriction and then binging on "forbidden" foods again in a damaging cycle.

Poor diet quality and high saturated-fat intake are often characteristics of carbohydrate-restrictive diets that are often recommended for optimal blood sugar control. Rigid meal plans designed for control within an extremely tight range claim to be a solution for treating diabetes. However, this method does not consider mental health or the diversity of people with diabetes, who each have unique nutritional needs.

Blood sugar control is only one part of living with T1D, and while I stressed over my A1c, the holistic approach to taking care of my body went unrecognized. "Eat whatever you want as long as you take insulin for it" was the wrong interpretation I had about food. Every day, I woke up to a body I was miserable living in, yet I continued to eat as if I was trying to hurt myself. All I focused on when I looked in the mirror was how much I disagreed with my physical appearance, without even the slightest idea that poor nutrition was affecting my digestive health, cholesterol, thyroid, and mental health.

Weight gain is common with intensive insulin treatment, but that does not mean a healthy body weight cannot be achieved while lowering A1c. Similarly, maintaining healthy blood sugar does not always mean taking more insulin. The relationship between *blood sugar, nutrition, exercise,* and *insulin* requires balance and thoughtful decision making. Understanding how one affects the others is not just a science but also a skill in self-awareness.

Weight gain does not always correlate with better glucose control. A study that closely followed the effect of intensive insulin therapy concluded that total insulin dose did not contribute to weight gain, but rather increased calorie intake was the cause. Frequent low blood sugars and increased appetite were observed in the participants. Overtreating lows with food followed by aggressively correcting highs with insulin is the most common cause of weight gain.[15]

People with diabetes should not have to choose between a healthy body weight or healthy A1c—both can be achieved. This balance will always push the boundaries of maintaining a positive relationship with body image, food, and mental health.

Insulin Does Not Make You Fat

Weight gain is common after diagnosis. Insulin helps the body recover nutrients and restore strength. The goal is to maintain a healthy appetite as blood sugars are maintained in a safe range.

- Weight gain results from excess calories and not from taking insulin.

- Intense hunger with drastic changes in blood sugar often leads to poor appetite regulation.

- Weight gain can result from overeating calories from any type of food, *not just carbohydrates.*

- When treating a low, eat fifteen grams of fast-acting glucose and wait fifteen minutes before eating again if blood sugar has not risen. I know this is much easier said than done, but it's the best way to safely treat lows while limiting calories.

- **Ghrelin** is a hormone that stimulates hunger. It increases during calorie restriction to prevent low blood sugars. When insulin has been taken, ghrelin can play defense by stimulating the appetite to prevent hypoglycemia.[16]

Calories, carbohydrates, and insulin have specific roles to play in fueling metabolism.

Calories are a unit of energy that each person requires in different amounts.

A carbohydrate is a macronutrient that provides glucose from food.

Insulin helps transport glucose to cells to be used for energy.

Insulin is not a source of calories, nor does it create body fat.

How do calories add up?

- 4 calories per 1 gram of carbohydrates
- 4 calories per 1 gram of protein
- 9 calories per 1 gram of fat
- 3,500 calories = 1 pound

The most common causes of weight gain in people with T1D include:

1. Improved conservation of ingested calories: *absorbing food better after diagnosis.*
2. Decrease in energy expenditure: *inactivity, slower metabolism with age.*
3. Hypoglycemia and overeating: *treating low blood sugar with too much food.*

From the moment of diagnosis, food takes on a different quality as something that must be calculated and controlled. To find a healthy balance, begin by noting personal challenges: for example, treating exercise-induced lows with too much food is a frequent challenge.

To solve this, we frame a specific intention to guide our decision-making, leading to better outcomes.

Now, an action plan can be developed to make better decisions using knowledge and skills. This helps you become an expert at reading your body!

Challenge: Exercise-induced lows.

Intention: Prevent overeating for treating lows during exercise.

Knowledge: Track and observe glucose and insulin records on days when lows are happening. Watch for patterns in food, blood sugar, and insulin adjustments before exercise.

Action plan: Adjust the timing of insulin and/or nutrition intake prior to exercise and observe the results. Repeat and continue to make small adjustments as needed until exercise-induced lows are infrequent.

Skill set: Become proficient in blood sugar management during exercise by making strategic adjustments to nutrition and insulin timing.

Weight management is not the most comfortable topic to talk about, but that's also why it's so important. When body weight is emotionally triggering, it can become a self-limiting factor that holds us back from exploring our potential. It's okay to feel burned out from the duties of diabetes, but using food to soothe emotions or exercising as punishment are not safe or sustainable habits. To feel better, we must intentionally take care of ourselves in partnership with diabetes, using a positive approach that targets emotional distress.

In addition to my lack of nutrition knowledge, there was one other factor that I hadn't accounted for, and it would be nearly ten years before I even considered it: *my hormones.*

The Period Puzzle

What's it like being a girl with T1D? Poor body image and struggling to feel normal often triggered unhealthy thoughts and reactive emotions. I wished to be invisible while I was treating my diabetes, as evidenced by hiding my hands in my high school locker while testing blood sugar and drinking juice in a bathroom stall so I could avoid being seen during lows. Diabetes was my burden to bear, but middle school was miserable for me for the same reasons it was miserable for every gal in that awkward stage of growing into her body.

Unfortunately, my middle school had a pool, and coed gym class included swimming. Everybody knows what happens when fourteen-year-olds get into a pool together: staring, blushing, whispering, laughing, and endless humiliation. I had bruises on my thighs from insulin injections, but nobody was looking at my stems while I was trying to hide the boobs that were coming in. Fortunately for me, there was always someone else having a worse day at the pool.

I was lucky compared to many of my friends, who started on birth control to deal with painful periods that sometimes persisted for weeks. I was thankful that my reproductive system operated as expected and my cycle was routine and relatively pain free. Statistically, less than 15 percent of women have cycles that are exactly twenty-eight days, and more than 20 percent have irregular cycles.

The funny thing about having a very manual disease is being grateful for the automatic processes that happen in working order. It's a knee-jerk habit to take note of things like this.

Thank you, period, for not making my life miserable . . .

Thank you, kidneys, for not failing me! And so on . . .

Those of us with T1D see what it takes to manage our blood sugar from the outside in based on careful monitoring and record keeping. It can be hard to cope when monitoring suddenly becomes a guessing game as to why blood sugar is fluctuating out of thin air. For numbers-focused people, it's especially unnerving when a natural function, like the reproductive system, throws blood sugar off track because we cannot control it. With random hyperglycemia, the only option is to take more insulin.

I had battled random highs without explanation for nearly fifteen years, and I was sick and tired of not understanding why until I finally had an opportunity to figure it out. I happened to be in the right place at the right time to put the pieces of the period puzzle together.

The roller coaster of erratic blood sugars and insulin adjustments can last anywhere from days to weeks leading up to the start of a period. It's easy to feel defeated when blood sugar suddenly becomes difficult to manage, leading us to harshly analyze nutrition and shame ourselves as if we are doing something wrong, but it's not our fault.

Being a girl with T1D is no walk in the park, and the phases of the menstrual cycle do not make it any easier. Adjusting hormone levels can lead to yo-yo feelings in addition to the sudden need to take more insulin.

The need for more insulin leading up to menstruation is not "a diabetic thing" but completely normal biology and nothing to be ashamed of.

I understand this can be really aggravating. However, a woman without T1D will make more insulin naturally. It is not wrong to take more insulin when the body calls for it.

Once I realized I was on to something with my own random monthly highs, I went on a mission to research the correlation between my inconsistent blood sugars that seemed to happen every three weeks and my cycle. For several months, I marked the starting date of my period on a calendar, and I realized my blood sugars elevated out of nowhere approximately ten to fifteen days prior to the start of my period. I also noticed that I was having lows the day my period started and up to two days later.

After researching the menstrual cycle and consulting with a friend who happens to be a gynecologist, I finally knew what was causing my marked symptoms: *that darn hormone progesterone and its friend estrogen.*

Fear not! We are capable of getting a grasp on this by tracking our patterns.

Approximately fifteen days from the first day of your last period, progesterone begins to increase for the purpose of preparing the body for pregnancy. Progesterone levels will drop if pregnancy does not occur. As progesterone lowers, estrogen rises, leading to the start of a new cycle.

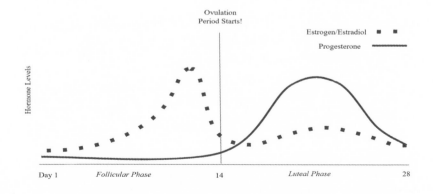

The hormone cycle demonstrates the ebb and flow of progesterone and estrogen. This visual provides evidence of when blood sugar may rise with fluctuations in hormone levels. Not every woman with T1D will experience hyperglycemia at the same time each cycle. Insulin resistance is temporary when hormones are high, with blood sugar typically dropping once your period starts.[17]

Follow These Steps to Investigate Your Hormonal Trend

1. Note the sudden need to take more than the usual amount of insulin.

2. Track basal, bolus, correction doses, and how you feel emotionally.

3. Record the daily total of insulin taken.

4. Continue to track this pattern each day that your insulin needs are higher than usual.

5. Note the day your insulin needs drop back to the typical rate.

6. Follow this routine for at least three months to discover your hormonal trend.

The steps above should help you devise a plan for making strategic adjustments with insulin, nutrition, and exercise. Please view this homework from the perspective of self-discovery, which is worth focusing on. I know that diabetes can be frustrating when blood sugar suddenly elevates. *I've been there! I'm still there!* I also know that sometimes it's easier to forget about a few tough days than to think about what's going wrong. However, when blood sugar is suddenly variable due to the natural order of the body, I find diabetes more forgiving.

What about Birth Control?

- If you are taking an oral contraceptive that delivers a constant amount of hormones through a twenty-one-day cycle, you may not notice that your blood sugar fluctuates.

- If you suspect that hormones are having an effect on your blood sugar, this method of tracking will apply to you. The only difference is that you won't have a period as evidence of hormone fluctuations.

- I suggest tracking the number of days your high blood sugars last and observing if there is consistency in the length of time from month to month. The goal of this practice is to tune in with your body and be prepared as well as possible to avoid low blood sugars.

It's not my fault that I don't make insulin, but it is my responsibility to understand my body. If only it were as easy as asking Google, *"Why is my blood sugar high today?"* But the body is not that simple. The best choice I could've made sooner would have been to embrace the changes in my body and try to understand what was happening. Learning to work with my challenges would have been wise, instead of pretending that it wasn't a big deal for my blood sugar to run mysteriously high for a week each month.

Figuring out my unique period puzzle gave me a dose of empowerment, but I didn't learn anything about it until I became a dietitian and shared an office with gynecologists. A combination of the right place, right time, and right people helped me learn how to manage this extremely important element of my body. Without this combination falling in line, I may have never had the opportunity.

TIP—Try using a calendar for crystal clear record keeping. This allows for easy tracking from month to month. I use a desk calendar to mark the first day of my period with a star and a line drawn through to the last day. Feel free to use an app or your phone to track, whatever habit makes the process easy and unforgettable.

On the Road Again

After the day at the beach with the manatee and declaring that I would start determining my own experiences in life, I first had to change the air. I had certainly learned what I didn't like about my job, my school, and the people I allowed around me, but what I wanted for my future wasn't clear anymore. Forcing this mismatch to align was never going to work, and the signs were everywhere. I completed a two-year degree and relocated to the opposite coast of Florida, where I couldn't seem to jump-start a career or make relationships work. My car became a magnet for bad luck, from parking tickets to flat tires, getting rear-ended, and then doing the rear-ending. I had a part-time job slinging martinis at a club when a new bartender showed up from a neighboring hometown in Minnesota. With his lighthearted energy, he represented the final ingredient I needed to embark on a new mission. I realized that it was time to take a load off, lighten up, and admit that my future was calling elsewhere.

I hadn't taken the leap to go home yet, but home had found me.

7

BREAK THE WHEEL

Don't tell me what I can't do

WHEN I TOLD my dad that I wanted to go to college in Florida, he encouraged me to become a dietitian since I was already "on the inside." I considered his advice for a few seconds before recalling that I was a terrible example and that no one should listen to me. Besides, the thought of being immersed in diabetes was appalling. Also, I'd never met a dietitian I liked; why would I want to become one?

This was Dad's way of encouraging me to learn how to live a healthier life, but I had to want it for myself. In high school, I had no hope for improving who I was. My plan was to move as far away as I could to *change* who I was. I had to take a detour and experience life on my own terms and make my own choices—the good ones and the character-building bad ones that work as catalysts for change.

It takes courage to turn attention inward and face the dark parts of ourselves. Dropping the frequency of truths we don't agree with and suppressing unfavorable memories are reflexive. It's in our nature to hide from things that make us uncomfortable and restrict our capabilities when we're afraid. Thanks to diabetes, I had become very in tune with my body. Although I spent years tearing myself apart, I had to face the pain and accept that I needed patience and the willingness to learn from bad days to improve my temperament.

Let it come, bring it on.

I chose to walk through the fire of self-discovery and enter vulnerable territory in an effort to create Lauren 2.0. It was a soul-crusher of a decision to move back to Minnesota, but necessary. The future was uncertain, and the United States was in the middle of a recession, but I was ready to start over. Working in healthcare seemed like a safe bet—safe was my new objective. I was exhausted from the risks I had taken, and I downplayed the ambitions I once had. Stability and health insurance were top priorities over traveling, meeting new people, and starting new hobbies.

I even had a new doctor, and I actually liked her. Big changes were already starting to happen.

What I needed to change was not going to happen overnight. Sure, I had the lifelong experience of living with disease, but the only way to become an expert was to enter the arena back where it all started. *Do what scares you the most* were words that tapped on my forehead from the inside. I felt the challenge in my bones, knowing intuitively that I swore to become the person I needed most.

Bold Decisions and Truth Injections

I decided to go back to college because I was utterly defeated by a career path in retail that was downright damned. Sometimes it was fun and creative, but most of the time I was talking people into buying stuff they didn't need to please higher-ups who never remembered my name. What a crappy deal that was, but I acquired some serious skills in sales that would help me own the floor at interviews I had coming in the future.

I looked over the dietetic program's requirements and conditions for taking the registered dietitian exam and decided it was nearly impossible. But for some reason, I felt like I was being dared to ignore a call of the wild. It was an innate decision to bite off more than I could chew and donate my sanity to a risk beyond reason. Line by line, I read through the application, required coursework, and the slim chance of getting an internship with a feeling of excitement. It was similar to when I moved to Florida on my own—it simply lit me up to do things that were hard and didn't make the most sense!

I applied a handful of prerequisite credits and was accepted. Just like that, off to college I went as an older student with real-world experience and a chip on my shoulder, but ready to hit the ground running. *Heigh-ho, heigh-ho, off to nutrition school, I go!*

I was not a great student, as evidenced by my transfer credits from "Beach U," and I've always struggled with multiple-choice exams. This was a bit of a problem for a brain wired like mine entering scientific territory.

What?! My A- in fashion history doesn't transfer? *Ridiculous!*

The C+ in government is acceptable? *That sucks.* I did not start off with a very impressive grade point average. *Are there any scholarships for underachievers?*

Historically, I only excelled in my two favorite subjects, history and English. As an unconventional student, creative writing and presentations were my thing. Not the typical top interests of a science student. The first two years were a struggle, but I held on to a satisfactory GPA by the skin of my teeth with unparalleled determination. The more the institution made me feel like I wasn't smart enough, the more I fought back.

Nutrition is the beating heart of diabetes, and I was going to master it one way or another.

My grades and attitude were hanging by a string until I reached the core classes, where I excelled in medical nutrition therapy. Even if the internship gatekeepers tossed out my B-loaded application, it really meant something to me that I earned As when it mattered the most. I refused to be intimidated while my peers who earned internships went on to train as carbon-copy dietitians, and I took this very seriously. The diabetes world needed a disruptor like me, and it electrified my competitive nature to shake up the standard approach.

I was emotionally invested in persevering as an expert who could correct the wrongs that had happened to me by standing on the other side of the exam table: *The sickly diabetic girl raises herself from the dead to become a health educator in the field of her diagnosis after being told she would never succeed either in health or academics. And the crowd goes wild!*

Fight Club

There are specific things in this world that awaken the temper monster that still lives inside me. These angry creatures collided in my final three semesters of the dietetics program. The expectations to speak a specific way and process information like a clone threatened my way of thinking. I was much more interested in learning how to communicate with patients than in food chemistry or having the ability to explain the process of coagulation in eggs verbatim on a written exam. Public health and classes that involved research interested me until the floor was open to discussion. I felt like I was wrong for wanting to call out current processes in healthcare or ask why patients are treated the way they are.

Current protocols for how patients are cared for in the health system as well as the opinions of students and professors revealed various undesirable interpretations of living with disease. Language that identified people as a disease rather than as living with one surfaced, followed by a few familiar labels: noncompliant, unmotivated, and poorly controlled. I found myself, yet again, in a position where I was expected to do what I was told even if I disagreed, and I'd already had a lifetime of putting up with that.

The pressure to fall in line was too intense without a little defiance to offset.

Ah, defiance. Hello, old friend.

If flippant was in fashion, I was a rebel on the runway with middle fingers held high. Group work and trying to bond with small talk for the occasional resume builder went fine until I shared my opinion on—*oh, anything*. I felt like the crass relative at the dinner table who told dirty jokes when she was supposed to say grace.

My desire to rattle the system became known when I stood out as the only student who took an alternative assignment after refusing animal experimentation. Once the experiment was over, several students cried in regret when their mice were "destroyed," wishing they had taken the alternative assignment. I was furious with the professor and saddened that so few of my peers chose not to stand up against something that was wrong. I went on to file a complaint with an animal rights organization that attempted to take action, but I knew it would be hard, if not impossible, for a little lionfish to demand change in a big university pond.

The challenge amplified when the director of the dietetics program announced that "B students" were not going to get internships. It was a blunt statement that jaw-dropped every student in the room before we had put in our first applications—no internship, no credentials, and this competitive program was designed to weed out less qualified students. Based on the number of available internships and the number of seniors competing for them, fewer than 10 percent would be placed.

Ah, here we go again, I thought. *Failure and disempowerment—my old roommates!*

Bring it on. I am not afraid anymore.

The odds were not in my favor, but I had to handle it with humor, or risk self-combustion. Most interestingly, my take-no-prisoners personality was foretelling, as I learned how much of an outlier I am as a patient and professional in the healthcare system.

The importance of developing counseling skills as nutrition educators was underestimated, as evidenced by having only one counseling class in the curriculum. Mock counseling scenarios and methods of delivering education were presented as simple and noncomplex. I wanted to shout, *"It doesn't work that way in the real world!"* In health education, a dietitian's ability to communicate effectively is the most important skill to develop, and I wanted to master it.

Realizing how low the expectations were took me back to Diabetes Island and how I felt like a miserable failure. It was painfully evident as to why I never understood food by the lack of emphasis on teaching skills. I began to speak out, as this was my opportunity to challenge the current delivery from a patient's perspective. Finally, I was feeling confident about something I understood better than other students competing for an internship. However, the director's statement hovered in the back of my mind, and I knew that GPA was all that mattered. And with that, I could have powered a lightbulb with my negative energy.

I Am the Thunder

My attempts at exercise would never be sustainable for two not-so-healthy reasons: working out was punishment (1) for eating too much and (2) for burning down high blood sugar. I didn't think physical effort was fun, nor did I expect to see results. Most days, I gave myself a guilty dose of encouragement to get up and move to work down my blood sugar, but the game changed when I threw down an ultimatum about controlling my temper.

I began to notice how anxious I was walking to class and how my thoughts raced on the way back. Mental unrest was a trigger point setting off my temper. Moments of calm came to me through music and nature, but somewhere on this pressure-loaded journey I had pushed aside nurturing myself.

I was raised listening to the blues, rock 'n' roll, '90s grunge, and a dash of heavy metal. Music that boomed with energy changed my mood within minutes, so I started making themed playlists designed to lift my spirits. This habit inspired the need for creativity.

Although I was always intimidated by exercise for fear of low blood sugar, I was compelled to test out my new and improved energy.

. . . and then a door opened to the university gym.

The discovery of indoor cycling classes was the perfect solution.

The university offered free group exercise classes, where the world of spin took me by storm. I was hooked after one hour of pedaling to top-volume music that I didn't even like. It wasn't boring or easy, but it was electrifying! The positive effect on my blood sugar lasted through the next day, which was all I needed to make spin my secret weapon.

A stationary bike gave me a sense of safety and control. I could test my blood sugar without stopping and keep my insulin pen and food to treat lows beside me with little fuss. Music also reminded me of home and summertime, even on days when the temperature was below zero.

Physical exertion matched with the energy of music was how I learned to let go of what wasn't serving me. I also had a good reason to plan meals methodically to improve my cardiovascular fitness.

As I pondered how to manage my anger with indoor cycling, I read a story about two cyclists with T1D that I couldn't get out of my head. Phil Southerland and Joe Eldridge started Team Type 1, which entered into the iconic Race Across America—an event that I thought was impossible with T1D—and the team won in record time!

Then came the jaw-dropping story of Kris Freeman, a cross-country skier with T1D who was diagnosed while training for the Olympics. He was the first to be diagnosed at this level in his sport, and though he had little support, he continued to train and compete. He refused to take no for an answer. Not even from the doctors who turned away from him.

I was starstruck. *Who are these mythical creatures?!* I never thought it was possible for people with diabetes to be more than average. These athletes were the examples I had longed to find, and they became my idols. Most wondrous of all, they were turning diabetes into a superpower. The message came through loud and clear to dig deep, dominate fear, and not let anyone tell you that you can't do something. I thought I could try to channel that energy into self-improvement and see what would happen.

Also at this time, I was beginning to build skills in the kitchen and care more for my body through nourishment. The old food rules were fading into the past, with positive results from non-scale wins. Food took on a completely different purpose as my energy lifted, with an attitude to match.

As my outlook on life elevated, I trained to become an indoor cycling instructor. The training made it apparent that my anger and blood sugar rode the same wavelength. The more consistent I was with exercise, the more mellow my temper. I enjoyed the physical work, and I certainly had the lung power to instruct, but the barrier was my lack of self-confidence. I wasn't very fit, and I secretly dreaded that dozens of people would be watching me from the front and back—thanks to the wall of mirrors.

Why do I want to do this again? To dominate fear!

My life's playlist was just as rebellious and passionate as my drive to succeed.

Despite all the unflattering traits I had labeled myself with, I wanted to become an instructor more than I was afraid to try. This was a ride-or-die mission that I put as much energy into as my studies.

The true determinant of confidence came down to the balance between nutrition and blood sugar. If I didn't have my protocol down to a science, I risked going low in front of everyone in class. *And I didn't want anyone feeling sorry for me.* The universe was dangling a carrot, and all I had to do was be brave and bold enough to wrangle it in, trust my instincts, and figure it out on my own terms. The goal was simple: maintain a healthy blood sugar range during my workout—no lows, no highs, feel good, become a badass instructor. This was where I could channel my anger—*I am the thunder!*

I began training myself alone in a dark studio, where I could focus only on my blood sugar and the music. Preparation was key. I planned to take extra care to get my blood sugar in a specific range at the start of training. I brought juice, glucose tabs, and granola bars to every workout. I had enough fast-acting carbs with me to go low a dozen times over again, but this was an experiment.

The first step was to cycle for thirty minutes without going low; I would break at twenty minutes, check my blood sugar, and continue, depending on where my number was. I repeated this process and tried several different methods between pre-exercise meal timing and insulin adjustments until I could ride for an hour with stable blood sugar.

Patterns emerged while adjusting to the variables, and it got easier as my physical conditioning improved. Eventually, I developed a protocol I could trust for any aerobic activity to prevent lows during exercise and avoid taking in excess calories! For direction on designing your own protocol, jump to page 170.

Training to become an instructor motivated me to study the relationship between exercise and nutrition for diabetes, opening a window of opportunity that I never expected. Mentally and physically, I was no longer afraid of challenging myself and presenting myself to the world. After becoming certified, I landed an instructor job and took over a Saturday-morning class that is one of the highlights of my life. Every week, I am privileged to ride with a community of amazing people to release stress and laugh by pounding pedals to the drums. Watching the participants transform before my eyes might be the greatest thing I'll ever accomplish. I see them leave class with more positive energy than they arrived with, and getting to be a part of that makes my heart thunder with happiness.

Outfox

In between trying to consider the opinions of others and teaching my cycling class, I contemplated my internship application. To prepare, I attended an open house at a hospital that offered a competitive stipend. This was a chance to meet the director and get a look at the competition, where forced small talk, fake smiles, and scanning eyes said it all. This was the Hunger Games of internships, and I had landed in the arena. GPAs of 4.0 radiated from every student except me.

Yet, I brushed my intuition aside and took a brazen risk when, truly, I didn't have a chance! I had hoped that my application letter would at least position me to interview where I might be able to talk my way in, but where GPA holds more weight than strength of character, I was not welcome.

Needless to say, the acceptance letter never came, and I was forced to get creative. I took interest in the idea of a distance internship, where I had the opportunity to design my own training rotations that would fulfill the areas of required learning. After a few months of tenacious networking across three states, I applied my plan to an out-of-state university, including the best sales pitch I could rally for why I'd make a tenacious dietitian. Fingers crossed that my information ended up in a better place than a paper shredder.

After six stressful weeks wondering if my future was crumbling before my eyes, the moment of truth appeared in my inbox: "Congratulations! You have been accepted into the dietetics internship program!" I jumped out of my chair, screamed into the air, sent the cats running and papers flying, then collapsed to the ground in disbelief. I lay there taking deep breaths, as if I'd crossed a finish line, until it dawned on me that the last four years were dependent on this acceptance letter. I had no expectations beyond this moment. I was sprouting like a field of greens.

And now, my life could start again. My stationary spin bike and I were off to the races!

This was my green light—no stop signs, no speed limits, pedal to the metal, coming in hot.

Ten months later, I passed the registered dietitian exam and became an official nutrition professional. Two years later, I became a certified diabetes care and education specialist.

It's okay if you're the type who wakes up to heavy metal, black coffee, and boot camp instead of meditation, green tea, and yoga. Discovering how to get into flow and live in the present matters. What we see as flaws that separate us can be entry points of motivation; living with T1D, my inadequate GPA, being unfit, and having knowledge gaps in nutrition, plus all the unpleasant experiences attached, were catalysts for change.

Imperfection made me who I am and a fighter down to my last breath.

Self-improvement has no timeline. You can go at your own pace even if it's not what other people are doing. Be strong in your convictions to make positive changes, and before long, either doors will open naturally or you'll have the tenacity to smash straight through them.

Sucker Punch

While studying dietetics, I was fortunate to get a job in guest services at a busy hospital. Before the first day, I was required to go through various health checks, including lab work and a review of health history, with the employee-health nurse. When my time came, it was revealed that I have type 1 diabetes. We discussed that my management was "well controlled" and my labs were healthy, other than a blood sugar categorized as high for a person without diabetes.

Unfortunately, the conversation didn't end there, and the nurse proceeded to give me an earful about complications. I nodded and followed along as if it were the first time I had been informed about the head-to-toe risks of my disease. If ever there was a time to quote Brené Brown—"If you're not in the arena getting your ass kicked, I'm not interested in your feedback"—it was now, but I held my tongue.

The nurse couldn't say anything that I hadn't heard before, until delivering this mind bender: "You know, it's not the lows that kill a diabetic. It's the high-low roller coaster that kills a diabetic."

Sucker punched right in the diabetes. *Please tell me I did not just hear that.*

A picture of the atomic bomb came to mind. Its cloud was billowing in my chest with AC/DC's "T.N.T." ringing in my ears. My inner voice was flinching in pain knowing that the first reaction that came to mind would have cost me this job with a police-escorted exit.

How could I ever forget such an inconsiderate comment? I was so sensitive to language used by professionals about diabetes that I never missed a thing. It was like sirens for offensive context were built into my temporal lobe.

The visit was abruptly over. I got lectured and left, but I was cleared for my new job.

Leave it alone, I told myself. It wouldn't be the end.

8

MOVE THE NEEDLE

Lean in to challenges with radical self-reliance

GROWING UP WITH a disease that is evaluated by people who don't live the same life can cause resistance. Being understood is a craving that requires honest empathy. When there's a disconnect between patient and healthcare professional, words and actions are easily misinterpreted as insensitive, trite, and impersonal.

As I was maturing, there was always something bothering me that I should have spoken up about, but all my appointments started and ended the same way: anxious going in, irritated going out. I never felt like it was the right time to talk about *me*, and I didn't want to uncover buried imperfections. Being labeled "uncontrolled" was so crushing. In my heart, there wasn't any space to talk about my greatest sensitivities, which bound my self-worth to a numerical value.

I need you to understand me isn't easy to say out loud. Getting real about feelings can be a desensitizing process over time when medical appointments feel rushed and regimented. Sitting down with a doctor who has an agenda doesn't make for an approachable "Can I tell you anything?" environment. Some people may feel inferior to an educated medical professional who may sound and look completely different, and it's hard to get vulnerable with someone we don't relate to. If it doesn't feel right to talk openly about vulnerable feelings, we instinctively suppress our thoughts to protect ourselves. Try as we might, internalizing the hurt will not make it go away.

Old wounds fester and affect our health in unforeseen ways when we bury them. Staying quiet about pain is not the solution.

If you're ready to identify your barriers, prepare to release them from holding you back. This is an important first step in creating a healthier space for yourself. Barriers don't have to be about diabetes, but you may find that the stress from worrying about them affects blood sugar.

Barriers I battled in the past had to do with my struggle to feel worthy enough to be healthy. I've had toxic relationships and un-rewarding jobs and doubted my intelligence. Once I decided that I deserved better and believed it was possible, I began knocking barriers down one by one with radical self-reliance. Calling out barriers is a way of recharging and taking a fresh look at what you are capable of.

Without bringing underlying issues to the surface and facing them, results will not be different. We are in the driver's seat and make our own choices, but nothing changes if we keep our eyes straight ahead and never turn the wheel. No matter how fabulous your support system, the best person in this world to advocate for you is YOU.

Take back your endocrinology appointment and decide: *This time is mine.*

Be fearless enough to work for your health. Discussing pain points is an opportunity to get to the root of the problem. Try to develop a mantra for during your appointments—something in the back of your mind that helps you stay focused on moving forward and getting answers.

Here is an example: "I am the commander of my health, and I will live my best life. Anyone who disagrees with my mission can step aside."

Advocating for yourself doesn't mean channeling a superhero, but on reflection, there's a reason my first role model was She-Ra. Every hero and heroine can teach us that goodness is worth fighting for, and in my lifetime, I've had to fight for my future. Wherever you are in your journey, living with diabetes or not, your health is worth challenging the world to care for.

You are your best and brightest advocate.

Getting the Most Out of Your Appointments

It's your body, your health, your future. Get clarity.

- Arrive early, not on time. Be the person who contributes to an efficient day.

- Be organized. Take inventory of the supplies that you need prescriptions for, letters you need signed, or school forms.

- Have a general idea of when your last pertinent checkups were—e.g., dental and eye exams.

- Set the agenda. Be assertive, honest, and direct, with specific questions you want answered.

- You can ask for external referrals to someone who can help with questions and concerns.

- Your clinic is a safe place to express anything about your physical and emotional health.

- If you don't understand what your care team is saying about labs or medications, ask for a clearer explanation.

Your care team wants you to succeed and supports you. If you need assistance in areas outside of the clinic such as safe housing, access to food, financial assistance, or community support, please make your requests known, and they will find the resources you need.

Action Words to Take into Your Appointment with You

Sympathy is not the same as empathy, and empowerment is different from self-sufficiency.

Sympathy is an expression of feelings, shared with concern for another person. This is different than trying to experience another person's life. Sympathy can be expressed for reasons that are not relatable but that show kindness toward someone's experience.

Empathy is golden. The feeling of speaking with someone who just gets you is the best. An empathetic person will try to walk in your shoes to know you better. It's a form of love to want to understand someone's experiences by sharing them too. Empathy is a sensitive practice based on trust and communication.

Empowerment is to give power from one to another. It can mean to allow authority, or the right to do something that wasn't in someone's power to begin with.

Self-sufficiency grows inside everyone. It's the part that continues to grow even at the worst times. To be sufficient is to be competent and independent with the ability to think for oneself and to make logical decisions.

I RECOMMEND RESEARCHING diabetes experts in your area to develop a personalized care team. You may find a provider who has diabetes that you'd like to meet. Send them a message. A compassionate provider will always answer your questions or direct you to someone who can. If your location is rural, telehealth may be an option as you broaden your search. Look into community events where you can get updates on research, technology, psychology, parent support, and a range of diabetes-education resources from healthcare professionals to peers with diabetes. *You may even see me there!*

9

LANGUAGE AND ATTITUDE

How we talk and think about disease could change the world

I N MY TIME as a dietitian, I've witnessed health professionals describe diabetes in a variety of cringeworthy ways. One particularly distasteful incident occurred during a Diabetes 101 presentation for a diverse health-systems office group. This should have been the perfect teaching opportunity to describe life with diabetes correctly—with esteem and respect for the individual.

However, experience rattles my nerves during presentations about diabetes, and I have high expectations. I have to ask myself what I'll do if I disagree—will I put my foot down and demand justice, or keep my cool, recognizing that the show isn't mine to steal? I often find myself deciding who to be situationally—the patient or the professional.

On this day, I chose to stay silent when a pediatrician described a continuous glucose monitor as "a nasty thing that a diabetic has to staple to themselves. . . . Who wants to do that?"

After picking my jaw up off the floor, I wrote this quote down. Spelling it out was the only thing stopping me from raising hell. Some may find humor in the pediatrician's words, or share the same opinion, but my trust was violated. I knew that my values were not going to align with this perspective on diabetes, and I wanted to blend in.

Just when I thought I had smashed the chip off my shoulder, it reappeared, uninvited.

Slamming medical devices that have immensely improved blood sugar management for millions of people is not a wise choice when there's someone in the audience wearing one.

A continuous glucose monitor, or CGM, is a device used by millions of people to help control blood sugar levels. This type of technology had been on my wish list for over fifteen years before it was available to me. Within a few months of using a CGM, my blood sugar had reached a constant, healthy level of maintenance, better than I had ever had in my whole life! *No staples required.*

I love the convenience of CGM technology and the range of information. Best of all is how continuous monitoring promotes self-efficacy and builds confidence in decision-making.

A CGM is placed on the skin with an ultrafast needle insertion that secures a tiny filament under the skin. The filament reads blood glucose levels continuously with minimal finger sticks. Fewer finger sticks and more visibility lead to better outcomes with insulin delivery. Useful data, including daily averages and time in range, provide a snapshot of how blood sugar changes over time.

Medical professionals who present information about chronic disease would be wise to assume that a person who lives with the presented condition is in the audience. An approach with compassion and respect is contagious, just as negativity and misdirected opinions can spread like wildfire.

IN AUGUST 2020, I had the opportunity to publish an article about why language matters in diabetes care on *Doximity*, a blog with a large network of medical professionals. I was elated at the chance to put my voice out there as a patient-professional. With evidence-based research and specific reasons why words matter for people living with diabetes, my work was published.[18] Within days, the article had over one hundred comments from a range of practitioners and medical students. However, what I saw in response rattled my hope for change within the medical system by the absence of empathy and denial of professional responsibility.

There were plenty of kind comments in agreement with using a positive tone and language that uplifts a person to their potential, yet they were mixed in with comments by physicians who stated their opinions in resistance to treating patients differently: "People are very sensitive these days," "Personally, I wouldn't care," "I'd like to see the evidence," "My patients don't want to change," "Why do we need to sugarcoat everything," and "How dare you tell me how to practice medicine" were among the regressive comments.

Several exchanges of vehement arguments between practitioners stood out. The most disturbing comments happened between a medical student and an internal medicine doctor who stated: "I'm happy to call any patient with diabetes anything they want if they keep away from the donuts, Blizzards, and Oreos."

The student replied, "I know you mean this comment to be funny, but as someone with T1D, I don't find it particularly funny. And I think I'd find it even less funny if I had T2D."

The only comment that took a personal dig at me was stated by a family medicine doctor: "I would like to have a job where I get paid to write such dribble." Another doctor replied, "The word you meant was 'drivel'—why so negative here?"

I did not expect the commenters to provide perfect examples of evidence for why my article needed to be written in the first place. Yet here they were in plain sight.

Showing a dauntless voice and calling on change in a profession rooted in traditional practices takes a thick skin. Sometimes while I'm writing, I wonder if I'm too sensitive and if it's all my fault that I've had a difficult experience with the healthcare system. Then I recall my behavior as a kid—the weight I gained as a result of turning to food to treat my emotions and feeling that it was my fault. I was the one choosing to hurt myself with sugar, not the doctors. They weren't trying to make me feel bad when they addressed me as "a noncompliant diabetic." In their eyes, they were offering solutions, but in my eyes, I needed something completely different.

With over 460 million people on the planet living with diabetes, and fewer than half meeting A1c goals, maybe it's worth taking a look at the patient perspective rather than revolving on the same wheel.

DIABETIC, NONCOMPLIANT, UNWILLING, unmotivated, poorly controlled, and *suffering* are frequently used words to describe a person or their actions in the diabetes world. These words can be seen and heard within a private medical record, in the pages of medical publications, and in lectures to describe people with diabetes. The widespread use of this language in the medical community gives permission to those in the practice to deliver the same tone. Professionals, family, friends, the media, and people who have diabetes have accepted these words as common practice.

In the past, I've called myself "diabetic," but I never liked how it made me feel. I would tense with avoidance, and I didn't want to be grouped with the diseased. Sadly, I was used to being judged and having to explain myself for what I was doing wrong. And I hated talking about diabetes just as much as I was burned out from constantly feeling like a failure.

The emotional depth of diabetes impacts motivations, behaviors, and outcomes.[19] Depression, anxiety, shame, and obsession with control are common traits of people who live by the numbers their devices display. Sometimes the effort a person is making to improve their health is not evident by observing data, indicating that facing challenges to see results is an inside job.

Shame can discourage a person from sharing their true feelings and cause them to hide struggles far below the surface. To be respected as whole human beings is crucial, so as to not lose sight of the person who diabetes lives with; diabetes is one part of a much larger puzzle. From head to toe to colon, the entire system is an intertwined partnership that needs love in equal measure.

Language lies at the core of attitude change, social perception, personal identity, and stereotyping.[20] People with diabetes are often viewed as complicated individuals who struggle to get on top of their duties and are often misrepresented as lazy or irresponsible. To the uninformed person, it can be easier to follow along with the stigmas of diabetes than it is to take the time to understand the person living with it.

Words are powerful and loaded.

Words can ignite and extinguish conflict.

Words that link disease to a person are emotionally triggering.

Words have the power to elevate or destroy with the slightest twist in communication.

Titles and labels can be awarded in praise or pinned without discretion.

Healthcare professionals may not realize the impact they have with words and tone alone. Even though our understanding of diabetes has expanded and treatment is more effective in the present day, judgment, blame, and misunderstanding of what life is like with a disease are widespread. The language of diabetes has focused on negative outcomes and fearful warnings related to complications that cannot be accepted anymore. The responsibility of changing medical and public perceptions of what living with diabetes looks like lies in the hands of the patient, who must own the way their story is told.

Self-Talk

For a long time, I tried not to listen to myself. The voice in my head was full of toxic messages that I tried to ignore, but they persisted until I decided to change my course in life. Even a string of good decisions didn't stop the inner critic that constantly reminded me of the things I wasn't good at, or had failed to do, or my perceived inadequacies.

Optimism was a rare feeling because I'd stopped believing that I was capable of more and deserved better. This was also the time when I pushed back against T1D and assumed that my body wasn't destined to age well. And that really scared me. Negativity destroys confidence and hope. Uncertainty and emotional pain directed my decisions until I changed my thoughts, which then changed my reality.

Rewrite Your Internal Dialogue by Building Personal Power

1. Find someone who is doing what you want to do; seeing what is possible drives inspiration.

2. Our words and thoughts inspire action; determine your experiences with positive self-talk.

3. Pain is a catalyst for the way we think; turn fearful thoughts into positive self-awareness.

4. Transform fear into wisdom by gaining knowledge in areas that accelerate self-sufficiency.

Inspired by sports psychologist Dr. Michael Gervais, host of the *Finding Mastery* podcast, https://findingmastery.net/category/podcasts/.

Self-talk is nourishment with the same purpose as healthy food: to provide positive energy.

How we feel about ourselves is tied to what we believe we are capable of. The desire to grow, learn, and feel healthy is a result of aspiring to achieve specific goals. A positive attitude changes the way we view the future, and attitude is what determines our life experience.

To get in **flow** with your internal positivity, choose an activity you can do several times each week when you are completely uninterrupted. Choose something that inspires happiness: painting, drawing, puzzling, gardening, reading, building, or fixing, to name a few.

To get in touch with your **purpose**, choose an activity you can do weekly that inspires the feeling of serving something bigger than yourself: volunteering with animals, reading to kids, donating your skills, or participating in spiritual activities that fill you with meaning.

To feel **connected** with others, spend time each week with people who light you up. If you are longing for a deeper connection, take a leap outside your immediate circle by trying something new. Connecting to others is about finding common ground, so expand on your favorite activities by looking for group interaction outside of familiar faces.

Limiting Beliefs

If you believe that you are only as good as the value of your A1c, then it's true.

Your thoughts are your reality. What you believe to be true is part of who you are, and your beliefs settle within your moral compass. The feelings, opinions, and core values that you hold dearest are demonstrations of your character. Family, personal responsibility, health, service, and kindness are a few examples of moral priorities. You can choose which values mean the most to you, and they can change based on personal experiences and influences. Trauma builds character; even as memories can be painful to recall, they are absorbed into every part of what makes you, you.

Our fast-paced environment is noisy, and it's loaded with messages we don't need filling what little clearheaded space we have. If someone treats you like your self-worth is tied to your blood sugar value, it's only true if you accept it. Persuasive opinions can settle deep within our psyche before we have a chance to think for ourselves. Even from a place of love, the people closest to us may not realize how much the words they say can influence our lives. The same holds true for what we allow to influence us in the clinic or the media.

Life with diabetes is a constant state of interactions that can cause limiting beliefs. They can be caused by an interaction with other people or a negative experience that holds us back out of fear, confusion, or an assumption not based on facts. For example:

1. You wanted to join the swim team but thought it was too hard with your insulin pump, so you decided that swimming wasn't for you and quit.

2. Grandma refuses to make your favorite cookies because she thinks you can't have sugar. Grandma cares, but she understands diabetes to be inflexible, with rigid rules about food. She believes that she is helping you by limiting your choices.

3. Your significant other doesn't want to tell their family that you have diabetes because it's too hard to explain. You are asked to test your blood sugar and use your insulin pen in the bathroom so no one will see you and start asking questions.

Limiting beliefs I've said to myself:

Exercise is too hard with diabetes.
I'm not pretty or in good enough shape.
I'm not smart. I can't pass chemistry.
Maybe I'm not supposed to be an educator since I don't fit in.
I want to write a book, but I can't face my memories.

Your self-worth is not tied to a number, a statistic, or the life experiences of others, and no one can tell you what to think. It may take a leap of faith and uncomfortable exposure to raise your awareness of how self-talk affects you. Determination and leaning into challenges can provide the support you need to get out of a negative mindset and begin stepping into the life that you want.

Desire is the foundation of all things. We can want and wish all day long, but desire sparks a flame that sets core values spinning into action.

Desire is what drives us to take chances and show bravery when we least expect it.

Desire gives us strength to put up with arguments and disagreements in order to get closer to the outcomes we are looking for.

Desire is a vision that is just waiting to become reality.

Growth Mindset

Two decades after T1D found me, I was hired to work as a dietitian in the same endocrinology clinic where I was diagnosed. Though it was not my goal, I had a feeling this opportunity might come, ready or not. Deep down, I had inner demons to slay, and the only way to salvation was to walk the halls where it all began.

Though the clinic had multiplied in size since I was a child, some things were still the same—a few familiar faces, even. However, I was on the other side of the exam table now, being trained to follow practical orders. Observing my colleagues test the obedience of young patients opened old wounds that festered with insecurity. The safest reaction was to play numb.

As I followed the protocol with lifeless enthusiasm, it became evident that yearly dietitian visits were often declined. Families got used to the standard checkpoint inspection about carbohydrates and found it to be an ineffective use of time.

How many kids in the last twenty years sat miserably in these rooms feeling just like I did but were unable to turn their lives around? was the tormenting question in my mind. I sat in my office chair like a bump on a log, pretending that I could do what I was told by following the standard suffocating approach.

But I couldn't. Under the surface I was a patient who embodied the scars.

My practice evolved the moment I chose to teach through personal experience.

When pertinent, I shared with families that I have diabetes. Having this in common bridged the gap of trust from patient to practitioner, and it completely changed the mood in the room from interrogation to invitation, with the unspoken motto *You can say anything to me, and I'll understand.*

Seeing myself in every young person with T1D and having the option to say "I have it too. I get it" fused our relationship, and I was honored to earn their trust.

Kids spoke openly about their personal struggles with food and exercise, which helped me ask applicable questions. In turn, families expressed feelings of fear and vulnerability that led to providing more effective resources. By changing the tone of the conversation, parents often expressed hope for their child's future rather than fear when they saw a grown-up example of someone living a healthy life with T1D.

I learned what others experience in my community, what it's like to be a parent of a child with diabetes, and how mental health is a persistent challenge. Walking in their shoes made me a better person, dietitian, and educator.

Connection is powerful when your experiences are aligned, but not everyone agreed with my methods. Several colleagues asked me to reconsider telling patients that I had diabetes and warned me to stay in my scope of practice. I was chastised for skipping business meetings to educate families, and I took lunch by myself to avoid conflict. To decompress, I used that time to work on playlists for spin class and to journal my frustrations to avoid expressing them verbally.

I was exactly where I needed to be, but it was a double-edged sword dependent on my attitude. It wasn't professional to let frustration do the speaking or slam my face into a wall, two things I had the urge to do regularly.

After a few years of working in stealth mode to avoid ruffling feathers, several of the doctors and nurse practitioners noticed my specialty. I became known as the sports-nutrition educator and started training other dietitians on how to broaden their conversations with families to connect diabetes holistically. One of the secrets to success for anyone working beside people who have diabetes is to become immersed in the lifestyle and build knowledge based on the human experience. Attending T1D community events, reading blogs, and watching trends on social media are distinctively important for making a personal connection.

Showing skills beyond basics with a down-to-earth approach opens the door for patients to connect and share personal concerns. Dietitians, in particular, are in a solutions-based position to offer education and resources to help improve lifestyle habits with out-of-the-box, creative thinking.

The old agenda was proving ineffective as the team of dietitians became more patient focused, inviting families to drive the conversation about lifestyle concerns, including nutrition, exercise, sleep, and stress, to expand the services we offered. The multidisciplinary approach oriented the clinic to work more effectively as a team to support families.

This was a time when I made invaluable discoveries about myself and the meaning of paying it forward. Increasing my knowledge of nutrition and exercise science became paramount, as food and physical activity were primary challenges not just for myself but for many people of all ages living with T1D.

PART TWO

NUTRITION

NUTRITION KNOWLEDGE

The Key to Prevention and Long-Term Health

If at first you don't succeed, become a dietitian

AN ACCUMULATION OF habit changes improved my life: going back to school to strengthen my knowledge base, surrounding myself with inspiring people, and leading spin classes. But above all, the prime game changer was how I chose to nourish myself.

I remember the last cheeseburger I ate, where I was, and who I was with. I declared, "This will be the last burger I ever eat," and it was. What happened over the next four to six weeks was out of this world.

At first, my only goal was to eat more leafy greens and fresh vegetables instead of meat, but I became more adventurous as my blood sugar improved. Whole grains and fruit made their way into huge salads that required half the amount of insulin I usually took for meals. Yet, I was eating twice as many carbohydrates!

I still ate tacos and casseroles, but instead of meat, I ate beans and as many veggies as I wanted, whenever I wanted. I wasn't focused on calories or weight loss even as the shape of my body began to change. Even my disposition and the way I thought about myself were becoming more positive.

Smoother digestion post-meal was the first sign. I stopped feeling uncomfortably full after eating, and my cravings changed. Fresh foods were starting to taste better in their natural form with little salt or added fat, and I was able to avoid dessert after dinner—that never would have happened prior to calling it quits on meat.

I was beginning to know the difference in eating for nourishment versus stress eating for emotional support. Quite frankly, this whole thing was weirding me out. I had no idea what was happening as my energy level increased and my blood sugar control made an unexpected turnaround.

Is this for real? I must be a study of one! Have I outsmarted diabetes?

Maybe I was a miraculous anomaly. Fair enough. Life had been one adventure after the next up until this point. The concept of eating more carbohydrates to improve blood sugar control may as well have been written in ancient Sanskrit, and nobody in the clinic was going to teach me that lesson. Eventually, the day I dreaded every six months arrived: my endocrinologist appointment, and I was due for blood work that would reveal the truth. I told my doctor that eating vegetarian was working out, and she could see from my glucose records that I was having way too many lows, so we lowered my insulin rates. She was supportive of my new lifestyle but was by no means an educator on plant-based nutrition, so she referred me to . . .

Duhn, duuhn, duuun, the clinic's dietitian.

I can't believe I agreed to it, but I was able to see the RD right away, so I went.

The experience was brief and painless, but useless, with two dietitians fresh out of internship. They ran through a checklist and spoke with me about carb-counting hummus for the duration of the visit.

About a week later, the lab letter arrived with my results and a handwritten comment by my doc that read, "Good results. Keep doing what you're doing."

Comforting but not exactly enlightening.

After a few months without meat and eating lots of whole-plant foods, I was no longer at risk of developing Hashimoto's thyroiditis, my cholesterol and triglyceride levels had improved, and so had my hemoglobin A1c.

This was awesome news! But what on earth was going on?

My choice to stop eating meat is probably the most important and pivotal decision I've made for my health. I wasn't trying to prove anything to anyone. I didn't do it for a social media post or under the influence of a public figure. I was simply testing a hypothesis to determine an outcome. I had no idea how well it would work until immersing myself in the science.

Dear Carbohydrates,

Diabetes welcomes you to the big show.

Hey, Carbs. I know it's tough out there.

I'm sorry for all the bad-mouthing, but a lot of people think you're a troublesome nutrient. I get that it's not fair, but you're confusing.

You identify as rice, broccoli, beans, and donuts at the same time.

It makes no sense to insist on being called by the same name in all foods!

How is anyone supposed to believe that carbs aren't the bad boys of diabetes?

Sometimes you drive blood sugar up faster than I can spell i-n-s-u-l-i-n.

At other times, you take it slow and steady, and I feel great.

Hey, Carbs. I need answers.

After the cost of insulin, no other topic in diabetes takes the spotlight of argument like carbohydrates.

Yes, carbs require insulin, but glucose is our primary fuel source. We need glucose to power every cell of the body, and the best part about carbohydrates is the vast range of choices. Vegetables and fruits contain carbs. Beans and whole grains contain carbs. Popcorn, pretzels, pasta, and tortillas contain carbs too. So do cakes, cookies, pies, donuts, and candy.

Our choice of carbohydrate matters most; how fast we absorb them during digestion and the timing of insulin are where all the magic is. Designating carbohydrates as either "good" or "bad" has little meaning once we understand the difference between simple and complex.

> Referring to a carbohydrate as "simple" describes a lack of nutritional complexity with the rapid rate of digestion. Simple carbs are often white as a result of processing; examples include pastries, candy, and syrup.
>
> On the other hand, "complex" carbs are digested more slowly because they are more whole and nutrient rich. Complex carbs contain fiber and often appear textured—foods like intact grains, vegetables, and legumes.

Carbohydrates get hated on by association because they are the primary reason for taking insulin with meals, but they also *unfairly* take the blame for causing weight gain. What I found to be the most important lesson about carbohydrates, and also the most frequent offense of inaccurate information, is assuming that every food that contains carbohydrates has the same effect on the body.

This couldn't be further from the truth.

The **glycemic index (GI)** was first established in 1981 as a method to help people with diabetes choose healthier carbohydrates.[21] Its introduction gives us some insight into the origin of carbohydrate counting. The concept of the GI is based on the rate at which individual foods that contain carbohydrates impact blood glucose levels. Foods are ranked from low GI (a slow rise in blood sugar) to high GI (a fast rise in blood sugar). Eating low GI does not necessarily mean eating low carb, but many of these foods contain fewer carbohydrates per serving, with the benefit of vitamins and minerals. We can classify them as having high nutrient value.

A Quick List of Where Foods Fall on the Glycemic Index

Lowest GI:

leafy greens, asparagus, peaches, blueberries, garbanzo beans, intact grains, and peanuts

Beans and bran fall between low and moderate.

Moderate GI:

bananas, carrots, sweet potatoes, high-fiber bread, cashews, and couscous

Pasta and instant rice fall between moderate and high.

Highest GI:

Cheerios, dates, watermelon, juice, french fries, teriyaki sauce, bagels, chips, candy, and toaster pastries

---

Eating a combination of foods across the GI scale can change the rules of absorption. For example, potatoes are considered high GI, but when combined with a cup of bean chili and a leafy green salad, the rising effect on blood sugar slows. Adding small portions of protein or fat can also slow the rate of rising blood sugar. The principle is based on nutritional value.

The GI is a simple guide to start with for anyone trying to make better nutrition choices. Between the concepts of glycemic index and carbohydrate counting, the quality of meals and nutritional value matter most. Even better, the common denominator in nutrient-rich foods is fiber, the nutrient that designates carbohydrates as complex, aiding in healthy digestion, lowering inflammation, and excreting toxins.

Sugar and the Brain

To get high on the GI, think of how it feels to take a bite of your favorite dessert. *Mmmm, I dream of Chicago Diner cheesecake . . .* Do you take a bite, close your eyes, and allow the decadent sensation to go straight to your brain? It may only last for a few seconds of bliss, but you quickly take another bite before the sweet vibes vanish.

We can notice how much sugar affects our mood and emotions when we eat mindfully. Sugar takes a one-way ticket to the reward center in the brain. Frequent reward stimulation is how we get addicted to substances that provide instant pleasure.

Dopamine lights up like Rock Fest when sugar arrives, and it's in our DNA to respond. We haven't evolved past recognizing that we don't need fast-acting energy all the time, but we gravitate toward it. Once we know how good the dopamine surge feels, we eat more sugar and desensitize ourselves to smaller amounts. This is a process of chemical reactions that teach us how to behave as goal oriented, but we can become addicts at any age as we learn how to associate dopamine with its source.

> Dopamine is a neurotransmitter that travels between nerve cells. It affects mood, memory, movement, and how we learn, feel, and sense reward. Dopamine release stimulates pleasure and addiction. How we choose to reinforce and repeat the feeling is innate, depending on the person. This is where drugs, sex, and rock 'n' roll coincide with food and exercise addictions. Learning how to limit the dopamine rush is the challenge. Music, meditation, and a few minutes in the sun, along with healthy nutrition and exercise, are a few methods of positive reinforcement that can replace unhealthy urges.

Added sugar is a worthless substance to consume for health. It exists simply for our pleasure, and we are a society that is obsessed with it—the average daily sugar intake in the US population is sixty-seven grams![22] The foundation of the Western diet comes with the price of convenience: fat and sugar are added to foods to make cheap, processed ingredients taste good—*too good.*

Fruit juice, granola bars, sauces, and dairy can easily triple a person's intake of added sugar beyond the daily recommended maximum of 10 percent of total calories.

For points of reference, 45 grams of sugar is 10 percent of 1,800 calories, and a 12-ounce can of soda typically has 39 to 46 grams of added sugar.

The best course of action is to avoid regularly consuming sugar-loaded foods and drinks. These foods contain the simple carbohydrates that raise blood sugar quickly. Ingredients listed as aliases for sugar are syrup, honey, and molasses. Sugar has dozens of different names, and the more we consume it, the more we want it. Once sugary junk food enters our home and locks onto our neurons, it's hard to kick.

The stress involved with high levels of dopamine and sugar overwhelms cells with too much energy. Too much sugar day after day damages mitochondria, the home of DNA and energy production. Losing mitochondria function accelerates aging and increases our risk of Alzheimer's disease and cancer.[23] Inflammatory stress and high blood sugar in the brain impair communication between neurons that misfire when they die off. These damaged signals change brain function, as proteins degrade into plaques that are difficult to break down. Cognitive decline is the long-term outcome of persistent high blood sugar, while surges of insulin cause more stress than brain cells can handle.

Break the Spell

Sugar addiction is an old friend of mine that tends to resurface when I least need it. Stress, boredom, seasonal affective disorder, and poor sleep are invitations for sugary stimulants. Sugar is around virtually every corner, making it a hard vice to shake, but there are strategies for cutting back without feeling deprived.

**Follow this pattern: replace before eliminate,
add before subtract.**

- Replace fruit juice with real fruit. Add water, coffee, or sugar-free tea. *Designate juice as a tool for treating hypoglycemia only.*

- Add berries or apple slices with cinnamon to plain oatmeal in place of brown sugar.

- Add fresh fruit instead of jam or honey to high-fiber toast with peanut butter.

- Replace dairy milk with zero-sugar, unsweetened plant-based milk.

- To expand salad dressing, add balsamic vinegar, lemon juice, or veggie broth.

- Choose unsalted nuts instead of honey roasted or sugared.

- When making smoothies, choose one serving of fruit, and add a cup of spinach or kale.

- When eating at restaurants, ask for dressing and sauces on the side for portion control.

Compare labels on these items to choose the lowest in added sugar:

- Salad dressing and marinades

- Spaghetti sauce

- Bread loaves

- Granola bars

- Cereal

- Vitamins

HISTORY OF NUTRITION IN DIABETES

The past teaches us how to nourish ourselves in the present

DIABETES WAS FIRST documented in ancient times as one of the oldest known diseases. Perhaps the oldest medical document in the world, the Ebers Papyrus was discovered lying with an Egyptian mummy dating back to 1552 BC.[24] This scroll reveals the observation of people who were parched with a painful thirst, lacking the ability to hold any liquids and dying from an unknown cause.

Sounds mighty familiar, doesn't it?

Even so, over three thousand years passed between the Egyptian observation and the published definition of diabetes. Then it was another three hundred years before the first insulin injection.

Several ancient Greek physicians had studied the advanced symptoms of type 1 diabetes, but they made little gains on causation. **It was determined to be a rare affliction due to the physically active lifestyle of most Greeks that adhered to a low-fat, low-sugar, high-fiber diet.**

Source: J.J. Anderson and D.C. Nieman, "Diet Quality—The Greeks Had It Right!" *Nutrients* 8 no. 10 (October 2016): 636, https://doi.org/10.3390/nu8100636.

Diabetes was named by Aretaeus of Cappadocia in the second century AD. The definition in his time came from the word *siphon,* to describe excessive emission of fluids and intense thirst.[25] Aretaeus had a medical mind far ahead of his time and was gifted in his descriptions of disease. Unfortunately, after the fall of the Roman Empire, much knowledge about medicine was lost, and superstition about disease set in. As a result, Aretaeus's studies of acute and chronic disease were lost to the world and not referenced again until 1554, when he was published. However, the absence of knowledge provided an opportunity for Arabic and Asian physicians to note the symptoms of diabetes—documentation that provided evidence of diabetes occurring across cultures.

Prior to the discovery of insulin, diabetes meant suffering until death by starvation. When diabetes was suspected, nutrition recommendations were designed to prolong what was left of a short life by cutting all carbs and decreasing calories. Organs began to fail as cellular starvation set in during a miserably slow death by ketoacidosis.

Once insulin was discovered in 1921, the nutrition protocol wasn't exactly liberating, but lives were now being saved. With insulin administration, diabetes was no longer a death sentence, but carbohydrates were still considered the problem. Meat, cheese, and eggs were primary recommendations because they do not contain significant amounts of carbohydrates and therefore do not break down to glucose. *I wonder what Aretaeus would've thought about this . . .*

In the 1930s, the "line system" was created for managing carbohydrates, and it evolved into the exchange system that is still in use today. Artificial sugar substitutes became popular along with the term *diabetic food* as the tagline for hospitals and cookbooks.

The goal of the diabetic diet was to take as little insulin as possible regardless of the nutritional benefit from carbohydrates. At this time, insulin was not as fast acting as it is now, and the design of meal plans was based on critical timing. In between meals, the goal was to avoid eating anything that caused blood sugar to rise, to

What's the problem with sugar substitutes?

Artificial sweeteners and sugar alcohols are sweeter than sugar but contribute little to no calories, nor do they raise blood sugar. The Food and Drug Administration declares them safe for consumption in reasonable quantities, but that does not mean everyone should use them as a method for weight management.[a] Research has found that when artificial flavoring is consumed frequently, it can cause a change in palatability of whole foods, increase cravings for sweets, and lead to overconsumption of nutrient-poor foods. This adverse effect depends on the individual, but limiting intake of sugar substitutes is recommended.[b]

[a] US Food and Drug Administration, "High Intensity Sweeteners," May 19, 2014, https://www.fda.gov/food/food-additives-petitions/high-intensity-sweeteners.

[b] M. Pearlman, J. Obert, and L. Casey, "The Association Between Artificial Sweeteners and Obesity," *Current Gastroenterology Reports* 19 no. 64 (2017), https://doi.org/10.1007/s11894-017-0602-9.

avoid the need for additional injections. Furthering the popularity of meat, cheese, and eggs, they were coined as "free foods."

Limiting carbs and eating "free foods" was the standard recommendation for the next thirty years, until a study demonstrated that people native to Asia and Africa had much healthier cardiovascular systems from eating starchier diets that contained whole grains and beans.[26] The findings were shared with the medical community in the US, and even though concerns had been raised about eating a diet high in saturated fat—*the sludge that takes down the heart*—it was not appreciated in the diabetes practice, where carbohydrate restriction had been the standard for decades.

Finally, in the 1980s and '90s, guidelines began to focus on fat intake. A reduction in saturated fat while increasing complex carbs was recommended to support the cardiovascular health of people with diabetes. Emphasis was placed on individual needs before uniform recommendations, *and I love the sound of this*, BUT—

SnackWell's hit the grocery aisles with one powerful processed punch to the gut. "Fat-free" junk food was all the rage in the early '90s, and SnackWell's stood out as the Pamela Anderson of the cookie industry. This wasn't a genius effort by food scientists to help people lose weight, but a ploy to convince people that quality didn't matter as long as it was low calorie. Eating fat-free cookies was marketed as a guilt-free solution to weight loss, *and we believed it!* We entirely missed the point that the type of fat matters and that all carbohydrates are not created equal.

Diet foods exploded onto the scene while the medical community went to research war, trying to prove which was worse for our health—fat or sugar? Food-marketing companies took advantage of this so that every new product that came out could lure in consumers with a catchphrase. This is the multibillion-dollar method that launched unregulated dietary supplements into gym bags and medicine cabinets.

We've traveled so far from the nutrition recommendations of the ancient Greeks to the era of the "diabetic diet." We've made space for artificial sweeteners, fat-free, sugar-free, anti-carb, high-protein, detox shakes, and fat burner supplements galore! Will we ever come full circle and finally recognize that the ancients were on to something about prevention?

For some incredible reason, we aren't learning from experience. Our eyes don't have to wander far from the produce section to see diet products oozing buzzwords from a feature display—*often near the pharmacy of all places.* As a society, we are still falling for it even though we have decades of evidence showing that restrictive dieting not only blows but doesn't work long term.

Somewhere between, *oh, just about the third century AD* and the mid-twentieth century, people forgot how to eat. *Or they were misled.* Losing interest in cooking for the convenience of drive-thrus allowed the food industry to make decisions for us. The correlations in the rising cost of American healthcare and the food system cannot be ignored as evidence of our poor statistics in health outcomes.

The cost of whole-plant foods increased, while nutrient-poor items have been dispersed across the majority of grocery store square footage. At the same time, meat and dairy consumption increased exponentially along the same trajectory as chronic disease.

Suzy

My first semester at college, I was willing to put forward the typical freshman gung-ho effort and involve myself in a number of different things. That attitude didn't last very long, but a conference about food systems was on my calendar. At the time, these topics didn't interest me, but as a newbie to the wider world of nutrition, I put on my smart clothes and showed up. Mostly, I was looking forward to the free lunch that you can always count on at nutrition-related events. This time, the stars aligned with clever symmetry to enlighten me on the science of vegetarianism in the form of a special messenger.

Once the morning lectures commenced, I piled up a plate full of roasted veggies, hummus, and falafel and sat at a table with other nutrition students. I spent the next few minutes estimating the carbohydrate grams I was about to eat and injected insulin at the table. This took a little extra time these days because I had to consider my workout after lunch, in addition to the mysterious lows I'd been having.

And the detailed thought process helped me avoid small talk.

Science-degree students do this thing where they try to outsmart each other in a type-A sort of way that is not for me. Instead of inviting myself into that iron maiden of conversations, I dove into my lunch and looked over the afternoon schedule.

Out of the corner of my eye, the chair to my right pulled out for a small, colorfully clothed, and energetic woman with a plate full of food. She glowed with something that I wasn't sure of, but I sensed that she was about to share it with me.

Nuts. I was going to get sucked into an entirely appropriate conversation.

She immediately asked if I was a student, and my answer was something like, "Yep, hoping to become a dietitian and work in diabetes, I think."

BIG mistake.

She replied, "That's great! I'm a dietitian and diabetes educator. How can I help?"

Here we go again. *Breathe, Lauren.* My protective conscience screamed, *Shield wall!*

As for my second thought: *What's this one going to say about what I'm eating?*

Shall we discuss hummus or "bad carbs" or some invisible rule you think applies to me?

I may have been green with freshmanitis, but I was here to become a dietitian. That meant the end of allowing clinicians to run their one-note nutrition agendas on me.

I collected my next words carefully and said in one big breath, "I've had type 1 for a long time, and I became a vegetarian and it's changed my life. I've never been healthier, and I came back to school to find out why because no one has ever taught me a damn thing."

I expected her to pick up her plate and run off, telling all her dietitian friends that I wasn't worth a box of rocks and should never be hired anywhere if I actually made it through the program. On the contrary, she didn't bat an eyelash and smiled as she took a bite of asparagus. She even snickered a little. Still, I braced for a snarky reply as I began to feel my cheeks fill with red-hot embarrassment.

This precious Tinker Bell look-alike in turquoise earrings with a pixie haircut turned to me enthusiastically and said in the sweetest of sweetheart voices, "I know what's happening to you—IT'S THE FIBER!"

Uhh, WHAT?! I spit all over myself. *Earth to Lauren! You wanted answers, and it's going down RIGHT NOW.*

"Yeah! Fiber increases insulin sensitivity. There's research about this. That's what's happening!"

Double WHAAAT?! Now I started talking a mile a minute.

"I've been eating this way for about a year, and I'm constantly decreasing my insulin levels and I can't figure out why, but my energy level is so good and I'm eating more than I used to! And I never thought fiber actually mattered. You're telling me I'm not a study of one and this is known?"

"Oh, yes!" Tinker Bell enthusiastically nodded, turquoise wings fluttering in delight.

It was not a myth that complex carbohydrates can improve blood sugar control, and there was much more to the story than that. She wrote down a few references for me to look into as she explained why evidence-based research is so important in the field of nutrition. Classic for an exceptional educator.

My ears and eyes were wide open, but still, she represented a lifetime of distrust. Although my emotional barrier was one hundred feet high, it was starting to drop a tiny bit as I listened. Something about her was different, and I needed more of that fairy dust as we continued to chat about fiber, references, and insulin sensitivity. All the things that existed in this mysterious realm of hers.

The lunch break was almost up, as the second half of the conference was about to start. I was not planning to stay, but I needed more from this amazing creature before I risked losing her forever.

"Can we stay in touch? I think I could learn a lot from you, if you wouldn't mind?"

"Of course! I'm the state representative of the Vegetarian Nutrition Dietetic Practice Group with the Academy of Nutrition and Dietetics. If you'd be interested in helping me at an event, I can let you know when the next one is."

I had no idea what she was talking about, but there was only one right answer.

"Yes, please! I'd love to."

"Okay, great! I'm Suzy and I'm vegan. Here's my contact information, and I'll email you. Bye!"

And she fluttered away in an aura of glitter and butterflies.

Did I just meet a vegan dietitian and diabetes educator who taught me more in a few minutes than I'd learned in sixteen years of having T1D?

This. Changes. Everything.

Suzy became my mentor and friend for life. I don't know where I'd be without her wise advice, and I'm so lucky that she chose to invest her time in me. We share the same feisty passion to improve the delivery of diabetes education, and she has a gift for appealing to even the most unbending opinions. "What Would Suzy Do" is on my mind all the time; she always supported my quest for self-improvement and encouraged experiences that advanced my practice.

She is the most likable, intelligent, kind, compassionate, and energetic of people, and she was the first in the professional diabetes world to earn my trust. What she doesn't realize is that knowing her helped me move past being an angry little girl and become a confident professional.

Does she actually leave a trail of fairy dust everywhere she goes?

Inarguably, YES.

It's a blend of pink and teal with a wee bit of Scottish whisky.

FIBER

My favorite F-word

THANKS TO SUZY'S references, I spent the next several weeks pancreas-deep in research, reading everything about fiber that I could get my hands on. The supporting evidence jumped out at me with two emerging themes: *fiber and insulin sensitivity; meat and insulin resistance.*

I was astonished to discover a variety of studies that presented evidence for plant-based diets across the lifespan[27] and evidence for improving and potentially reversing type 2 diabetes.[28] Individual experiences were similar to mine, even with a different type of diabetes. I began to understand how my new food choices improved the efficiency of my digestion and led to an energy boost. The healthier environment in my gut had direct ties to mental clarity and blood sugar control. And I was having fewer highs because fiber digests slowly, causing glucose to enter the bloodstream at a slower rate.

Now it made sense why my doctor had decreased my insulin rates.

The similarities in what I read and how I felt were starting to make sense. Although I had no chance of reversing T1D, I was capable of increasing my insulin sensitivity by choosing the right foods. Essentially, my body required less insulin with fiber-rich foods, and my insulin bill went down as a result.

Fiber was literally saving me money. *Holy fireworks. Let freedom ring!*

It became crystal clear that trading in animal products for whole-plant foods was the simple solution to insulin sensitivity. Finally, I understood what happened to me.

I want to be clear about my position on carbohydrates: I am not a high-carb advocate any more than I am a low-carb advocate. Nutritional quality and individual needs matter most. We all deserve to know how many grams of carbohydrates, fat, and protein our body needs to be healthy. And this is where the often-turbulent debate on dieting for blood sugar control fires up.

There is a wide range of choices between low carb and high carb where we can have a healthy relationship with food, but there can be pressure in the diabetes community to declare ourselves as one or the other.

But we don't have to.

We only need to make a commitment to nurturing our physical and mental health.

Insulin Resistance

Prior to becoming a dietitian, I thought that insulin resistance was only an issue for people who had type 2 diabetes because they still make insulin, just not enough. *Oh, man, was I ever wrong.* Understanding insulin resistance in type 1 diabetes is important because we can improve it.

And I am living proof that nutrition is the key.

Research shows that insulin resistance is caused by intramyocellular fats in the bloodstream. How does this happen?

1. Fatty acid particles accumulate in the bloodstream.

2. Muscle cells store the excess fat, making it difficult for glucose to enter cells.

3. Glucose remains in the bloodstream, leading to high blood sugar.

4. Fatty acid accumulation causes a demand for more insulin when blood sugar is high.

Blood sugar elevates and insulin needs increase when fat clogs up the pathway for glucose to enter cells. Small particles of fat are like cars on the highway that clog traffic, resulting in elevated cholesterol and blood pressure. Cutting carbs can cause rapid changes in blood sugar, which may look like a solution; however, nutrition quality speaks the loudest when it comes to long-term results.

The reason I became more insulin sensitive was due to several factors:

- A wider variety of anti-inflammatory foods, spices, and herbs in my diet.

- Improved gut health and digestion from eating vegetables and beans daily.

- Eliminating meat, dairy, and eggs and consuming protein from plants only.

- Replacing saturated animal fats with nutrient-rich nuts, seeds, and avocados.

- Consistent high-fiber meals that led to more predictable blood sugar outcomes.

- Increased aerobic exercise due to having more energy and confidence.

Improving my metabolism could be owed to the addition of nutrient-rich foods and regular exercise while decreasing fat, hormones, and antibiotics from animal products.

I had upgraded my mechanics, similar to restoring a classic car!

Increased insulin sensitivity and metabolic efficiency go together like peas and carrots. Just like insulin resistance and inflammation burn together like grease and alcohol. Inflamed tissues result from damaged cells that are in need of repair. The more time and resources our body spends fixing cellular damage, the more rapidly we age. The unhealthy effects of chronic inflammation are less noticeable over time as the body adapts to joint stiffness, sore muscles, fatigue, and brain fog. These warning signs can become undetectable even as the body suffers cellularly from high-fat, salty, sugary, and nutrient-poor processed foods.

This explains why I struggled with the typical diabetes diet plan; I limited my nutrient intake by restricting complex carbohydrates. Cravings for simple carbohydrates were the result of not eating enough nutrient-rich foods, while my body was forced to adapt to an inflammatory state and high blood sugar. *The high-protein and high-fat foods I was advised to eat may have had little effect on blood sugar, but they hurt me everywhere else.*

Interestingly, the problems and solutions to living healthy come from the same place: our food choices.

I was ecstatic about putting this plant-based puzzle together, but underneath the elation, I was awake in the middle of the night, pillow punching with rage, pissed.

How many doctors and dietitians had I seen over the years?

How many hours had I spent listening to the same lesson on nutrition?

Why had I never heard anything about this research?

At any point, did someone try to talk to me about it and I ignored them?

The positive changes happening to my body were real, with scientific proof, but it was up to me to figure that out. If I had met Suzy sooner, maybe I could have avoided the anger, self-hatred, and frustration. At the very least, I would have avoided thousands of calories in juice, granola bars, and peanut butter sandwiches to treat low blood sugars.

ARRRRRGH! I'm seeing red. Quick! Say the mantra:

Go teach spin—go teach spin—go teach spin—don't get a speeding ticket.

Fiber for Prevention

The Academy of Nutrition and Dietetics states that "the mean intake of dietary fiber in the United States is 17 grams per day with only 5% of the population meeting the Adequate Intake."

A series of systematic reviews that considered the fiber intake of 4,635 adults found that reduced risk of disease is greatest with fiber intake of at least 25 to 29 grams per day. And even higher consumption of fiber could offer greater benefits of preventive healthcare. This data compiled from 185 prospective studies and 58 clinical trials provides evidence for "reduced body weight, lowered cholesterol, reduced risk of coronary heart disease and incidence of diabetes, with higher intakes of dietary fiber."[29]

A review of evidence determined that intake of fruits, vegetables, whole grains, nuts, and legumes reduces the risk of chronic diseases and premature mortality: "The current results strongly support dietary recommendations to increase fruit, vegetable, whole grain, and nut intake for coronary artery disease and stroke prevention." It concluded that "diets high in plant foods could potentially prevent several million premature deaths each year if adopted globally."[30]

The findings on the benefits of fiber are significant, while the fresh take on guidelines encourages complex carbohydrates, decreased saturated fat, and a patient-centered approach. The culture shift from *what is* the "standard American diet" toward what *could be* demands new and improved methods of education that focus on individualized nutrition needs and flexibility.

So, where do we start? We simplify our food choices and prioritize nutrient density.

View whole-plant foods for what they are: nutritious and colorful solutions for prevention and supportive of a healthier lifestyle, with or without chronic disease.

Fiber Guides Healthy Carbohydrate Choices—Tips and Tricks

1. Begin with a grocery list organized by day of the week and with specific meals, like a menu. Keep it simple—meals can be repetitive! This helps ensure that you bring home exactly what you want to eat.
2. Think about fiber-rich foods categorically; choose beans, veggies, whole grains, and fruit as the primary foundation when creating your weekly meals and snacks.
3. Upgrade your whole grains. Expand your choices to include wild rice, quinoa, barley, buckwheat, sprouted grain, corn, brown rice, and couscous for versatile options. Choose a serving of whole grain as a base for a veggie bowl or stir-fry. Use high-fiber tortillas to make breakfast burritos and veggie wraps. To put a spin on the classic PB and J, turn your sandwich into a higher-fiber roll-up!
4. Replace meat with beans. Drain and rinse a can of beans

in place of half a pound of meat to increase fiber while decreasing saturated fat. Add low-sodium taco seasoning, salsa, or garlic and black pepper to kick up the flavor. Having baked potatoes for dinner? Top them with beans, salsa, avocado, and a dash of enchilada sauce for an extra punch of fiber-rich nutrition.

5. Step up your greens. Leafy salads and raw veggies don't have to be boring! Get creative with vegetables by using the flavors you already love with your preferred texture. Try using your favorite dressings and marinades, or spices and herbs, with steamed or roasted veggies. Frozen and canned veggies are convenient and healthy—just be sure to strain and rinse canned products before flavoring to remove excess salt.

6. Choose colorful foods. There are waves of colors in the fresh-produce section, but frozen fruit is always in season. Blend berries into green smoothies; add mixed fruit to oatmeal or bran cereal for a fast, fiber-rich breakfast. Apples, pears, oranges, and carrots brighten up a kitchen bowl any time of the year. Strawberries and pineapples are great for snacking and can be included in both salads and on pizza. When expanding your range of choices and how you eat fruits and vegetables, you'll discover more ways to eat in color, filling every cell of your body with high-quality, nutrient-rich energy!

The golden rules of increasing fiber are chew slowly, cook thoroughly, avoid gulping, and drink plenty of water throughout the day. Fluid keeps fiber moving as it bulks in the digestive tract, picking up toxins along the way to the ultimate exit. Cramping and gas are normal and temporary as the environment inside your gut strengthens and improves immunity with a collection of new and improved bacteria.

Labels—Grams in Weight vs. Grams of Carbohydrates

Fiber lives within the carbohydrates listed on a food label—just below total carbohydrates and above sugars or added sugar.

A serving of food has a total weight in grams. For example, a granola bar is a single serving of food in one package, whereas a box of crackers will have several servings per package. The label may say twelve crackers per serving and six servings per box. This means there are seventy-two crackers in the entire box (assuming they aren't broken or crumbled to bits).

Carbohydrates account for some of the total weight of a serving, *but not all of it!*

Example: one of my favorite granola bars weighs forty-five grams, and the total carbohydrate content is twenty grams. It's important to understand the difference to avoid mixing these numbers up—especially when counting total carbohydrates for the purpose of dosing insulin!

Nutrition Facts

Serving Size: 1 bar (45g)
Servings Per Container: 12

Amount Per Serving

Calories 190   Calories from Fat 70

	% Daily Value*
Total Fat 8g	**12%**
Saturated Fat 4g	**20%**
Trans Fat 0g	
Cholesterol 0mg	**0%**
Sodium 85mg	**4%**
Total Carbohydrate 20g	**7%**
Dietary Fiber 4g	**16%**
Sugars 11g	
Protein 10g	**15%**

Vitamin A	0%	•	Vitamin C	0%
Calcium	2%	•	Iron	8%

* Percent Daily Values are based on a 2,000 calorie diet. Your Daily Values may be higher or lower depending on your calorie needs.

	Calories	2,000	2,500
Total Fat	Less than	65g	80g
Saturated Fat	Less than	20g	25g
Cholesterol	Less than	300mg	300mg
Sodium	Less than	2,400mg	2,400mg
Potassium	Less than	3,500mg	3,500mg
Total Carbohydrate		300g	375g
Dietary Fiber		25g	30g
Protein		50g	65g

Calories per gram: Fat 9 • Carbohydrate 4 • Protein 4

Daily fiber minimums per day	
Age (in years)	**Grams of fiber/day**
1–3	19
4–8	25
Girls 9–13	26
Boys 9–13	31
Girls 14–18	26
Boys 14–18	38
Women 18–50	25
Men 18–50	38
Women 51+	21
Men 51+	30

Please read nutrition labels or use a food scale for the most reliable measurements.

A dozen healthy choices, portion size, and estimated fiber content		
Black beans	1 cup	15 grams
Garbanzo beans	1 cup	12 grams
Soybeans	1 cup	15 grams
Blackberries or raspberries	1 cup	8 grams
Quinoa, wild rice, bulgur	1 cup	3–8 grams
Oats	½ cup	4 grams
Leafy greens	1 cup	4–5 grams
Flaxseed	1 ounce	8 grams
Acorn squash	1 cup	9 grams
Broccoli, Brussels sprouts, cauliflower	1 cup	5–6 grams
Apple, orange, peach, pear	1 fruit	3–6 grams
Potatoes	5 ounces	3–4 grams

Subtracting Fiber Guidelines and "Net Carbs" for Insulin Dosing

Researchers have looked into the properties of fiber to try to set a standard for meal insulin dosing, but there is no one rule. The choice to subtract any amount of fiber from carbohydrates is up to the individual, but notice that "net carbs" is not a scientific term. It was invented by food manufacturers, and it has absolutely no value to those of us who take insulin.

Everyone digests and absorbs food differently. This can depend on age, the environment inside the gut, and activity level. No two stomachs are alike! Since we are unique digesters, it's important to determine which food sources of fiber are most compatible with our system and blood sugar goals.

For best results, be sure to take your meal insulin before eating. This will give insulin a head start on absorption before glucose enters the bloodstream. If blood sugar is spiking higher than expected, it may be beneficial to buy time and dose a few minutes earlier than usual. And it's always a good practice to double-check the carb count to ensure accuracy.

A note on continuous glucose monitors: be patient. CGM devices allow us the convenience of watching our blood sugar at all times, but remember that blood sugar always rises when we eat. This happens to all people and it's normal. If it appears that your blood sugar is rising farther out of range than you are comfortable with, ask yourself if you dosed correctly before giving more insulin. Impulsive dosing within the time that insulin is active is also known as "rage bolusing," as insulin stacks, often leading to hypoglycemia.

DIET CULTURE
AND DIABETES

Focus on healthy practices for long-term results

IN SIMPLIFIED TERMS, I was *eating myself healthy*. I wasn't fixated on the scale or how fast I could shrink, although it felt much better to have less pressure on my stomach, as the effect of lowering inflammation in my tissues was noticeable. I was looking for healthier blood sugar control with a total-system approach, rather than trying to follow a diet that only targeted a lower A1c.

When it comes to dieting and the culture of weight loss, we know that rigid diet plans and pay-per-meal programs sometimes work. Yet we aren't keeping the weight off. Very few of us with beating hearts enjoy being told that we can't eat something.

It's entirely different when we choose not to eat something for a greater purpose.

When we are told what to do rather than taught a skill that allows us to choose for ourselves what's acceptable, we may not follow the rules for long. Diets are always rules driven, and no one commits to dieting with the mindset that it'll last forever.

"Just until I lose ten pounds," or, *"Once I fit into my skinny jeans again."*

Then the diet's off and the weight comes back on.

We walk a very fine line with our use of food for both pleasure and punishment. It's not an excuse that we have lots of external influences like work, commuting, and home life that cause stress. When blended with emotional turmoil, our reactions often lead to medicating with food and taking drastic measures to renounce habits as fast as possible. Time is precious in our modern world, and sometimes the proactive approach leads to unhealthy solutions. Rigid meal programs are tried and failed, while *diet* remains an unfavorable four-letter word, setting someone back in both motivation and cash.

Most of us can admit that we've purchased something because a beautiful person influenced us to do so. I can admit to being duped by photos edited to the wrinkle-free nines.

The marketing concept is simple: hire a gorgeous person to endorse a product and watch it sell. It doesn't matter if the product actually works. Diet-supplement companies love to use terms like "scientifically proven system"—fancy words formatted to earn our trust. Then a marketing team gives a simple product an ego injection of unicorn dust before millions of units hit the shelves. And that's how we fall for unregulated and mediocre products.

Fad-diet pyramid-marketing industries thrive on our lack of patience and our desperation. The best customer for any multilevel marketing company is a frustrated person strapped for time. The internet floods our senses with conflicting literature from unreliable sources: whoever has the loudest hashtag gets the most attention— and that's about as scary as misleading information gets.

Trendy diets have a few things in common:

- Short-term promises that thrive on insecurity and poor self-image.

- Well-marketed and profitable images sold by a model or celebrity.

- Nutrient restriction, often extreme and unsustainable.

- Unregulated claims and promises supported by biased evidence.

While it's madness that we continue to fall for the same diet scheme, the information age we live in provides a platform to repackage similar ideas. Mediocre sources with the power to influence scrollers on how to eat and what to buy are taking health seekers down one by one as they rapidly absorb information.

We are wise enough not to believe everything we see, but the serious question is *Who can we trust for health information?*

An exasperated phrase I often hear from people seeking to lose weight is "I'm so sick of conflicting information about nutrition that I don't even want to eat anymore." They've been inundated with dieting advice from neighbors, personal trainers, and online influencers who encourage crash tactics via scroll-topia, while in real life, donut day at the office, birthdays, weddings, and trending cupcake recipes attack the appetite from every angle. Toss in a long workday that concludes in a miserable commute that steers a stressed-out person straight into a fast-food drive-thru.

To add to the stress of dieting, there are more wearable devices on the market than places to wear them. In our scheduled lives, we've come to feel like we can't be well without the latest gadget. Now, being healthy feels like a chore, with added tasks that cost time as well as money. One must track sleep, food, exercise, water intake, and bowel movements to reach a goal. All this information is great, but totally arbitrary if we don't know what to do with it.

Although we have access to an enormous amount of information, every gadget under the sun agrees on one thing: you must do the work yourself if you want to see results.

What's the best way to avoid becoming a lifelong dieter? *Stop being one.*

Our bodies send very clear messages all the time. Feelings of intoxication, confusion, and lethargy are warning signs of a diet gone wrong. Think of these symptoms as internal check-ins and reminders that our bodies do what is necessary to keep all systems going strong, even under stressful circumstances. The more often we push our metabolism to operate under drastic conditions, the less we support long-term results.

Weight gain after repeated crash dieting is evidence of your metabolism warning you to check yourself. Persistent restrictive dieting patterns can inhibit our ability to lose body fat or keep it off as we age. It can even accelerate aging.

Metabolism favors nutrient value, consistency, and longevity. With time, knowledge and commitment to healthy habits pay off in the form of cash we aren't spending on diet supplements, prescriptions, and urgent care.

When we understand that our energy needs are unique and how to fuel properly, we stop allowing snake-oil hack science to cloud our vision.

The food industry is in the big leagues of bias and contradictory information; to them, diet *is a four-letter word—as in c-a-s-h.*

The business of nutrition is not the same as the practice. When doing your own reading of scientific studies, I urge you to look up the bio of the first author listed and check the bottom of the article to see if it was funded by any particular industry that may have swayed outcomes. Scientific research is often funded by a motivated party that expects outcomes to point consumers in the direction of their products—of the industry, supplement, and pharmaceutical kinds.

And it's happening in diabetes.

Studies that select motivated individuals rather than using random selection often have biased results. The design of this type of study is to prove the purpose correct. Otherwise, it probably wouldn't be published. This isn't to say that every study with motivated folks is wrong or bad, but I encourage you to research with caution. Email experts in the field you are researching. Take notes and self-advocate.

Here's my "take a deep breath" recommendation: *look into opposing research, as much as it drives you nuts. Understanding why people are motivated to do things differently than you is a respectful, high-road approach, and that matters in our connected world. It's better to attempt to find common ground with those we disagree with than leave huffing with anger and further division.*

Personal responsibility is one unwavering line drive toward a healthy body and mind, and it's up to the individual to choose this path for themselves. It takes a leap of faith to leave dieting behind and choose long-term habits over short-term, get-fit-quick schemes.

Pills before Skills

Going to the doctor's office isn't anyone's idea of a good time, but it's become part of our culture to seek solutions via a quick-fix script. Practicing unhealthy habits, waiting until a problem presents, and becoming dependent on pills isn't anyone's goal, but we've been conditioned to accept this conclusion. Humans aren't particularly skilled at adapting to sudden change. We are often accustomed to problems that come on slowly and are easy to ignore until a worse problem presents.

This pattern is common in the development of chronic diseases that are related to lifestyle choices.

High blood pressure and high cholesterol are conditions that often require medication. Swallowing a pill is minimally invasive and allows a person to carry on with usual daily habits. People are capable of lowering their blood pressure and cholesterol without pills or in combination, but why bother to change if medical practitioners skip the part about lifestyle education?

In Western medicine, prescription drugs are a frontline defense. Chemical solutions bypass lifestyle conversations, saving time for everyone involved. A prescription might be accompanied by paperwork with a short list of suggestions. A few of the common DIY recommendations are 5 percent weight loss, exercise 150 minutes per week, and eat more fruits and vegetables. Simple, right?

In reality, there isn't a standard nutrition handout with enough magic in its graphics to feng shui someone's health into perfect order. The solution begins with a relationship that treats the whole person, not just the disease or dysfunction. Treating the person helps to determine what lifestyle habits put them at risk. Solutions are discussed collaboratively as goals, and the order of priorities is determined by the person. This may or may not require pharmaceuticals, but it most definitely will require trust and sensitivity.

Five percent weight loss requires support and skill building. Eating more fruits and vegetables calls for strategy and creativity. Exercising for 150 minutes per week involves committed effort. *How does a patient get anywhere without the right support?*

What do general weight-loss recommendations mean to the person living in a small town with six fast-food restaurants, a gas station, a liquor store, a pharmacy, and a casino on the main drag, while the closest grocery store is twenty-five miles away? *Not much.*

This person will leave their appointment to carry on with the same habits, but with an additional detour to the pharmacy before heading home.

All they gained was a knowledge deficit and a bottle of pills.

Imagine what it might be like to walk in the shoes of this person, who will continue to live each day on the same wheel of hopelessness, returning to appointments quarterly to refill medications and leaving with the same directive every time. They are not asked about barriers or what kind of life they want to live, and they have little knowledge of how to change course on their own.

Expectations set at the lowest bar prevent patients from developing skills to help themselves. And although we must choose to take action, without encouragement from primary care professionals, we are stuck playing defense with our health.

One truth screaming loud and clear is that people with chronic disease want to live better, free of pain, and they are willing to make some effort. The problem comes when they seek counsel that points them down the wrong path, with unreasonable rules to follow, little support, and no guide by their side. Equally unjust is the advice of alternative practitioners who claim to cure through costly tests and dietary supplements in protest of standard medical practices.

Chronic conditions are not often localized. A condition like metabolic syndrome is hard on the heart, immunity, hormones, and digestion. This can lead to high cholesterol, frequent sickness, irritable bowels, hypothyroidism, and type 2 diabetes. A pill can't take away obesity as quickly as it can lower cholesterol, but a prescription is the easiest solution. At the same time, lifestyle conversations drop off the clock because they are the most time- and resource-consuming interventions.

When appointment time is over for someone with metabolic syndrome, they may be provided a prescription and perhaps a food list. Maybe it's a colorful handout explaining how to build a meal on a plate. Maybe a scribbled note reads something like "Eat foods from this list and come back in three months to check your weight." *How motivating.*

A positive experience is like riding a tandem bike: two people working together to make the wheels move smoothly. A negative experience might look like ping pong: firing back at each other until one opponent loses. An experience like ping pong in any clinical setting is the opposite of productive or relationship driven. Sadly, accounts like this have been shared with me from coast to coast by people who feel stuck and unheard. Each of them has the common goal to develop skills to be more self-sufficient. However, the most significant barrier they have in common is their doctor.

Know that doctors are in service to their community.

The patient doesn't take a bow of subjection for treatment.

Feeling heard and cared about is a priceless necessity that inspires positive health outcomes.

This is the human factor, and it means everything.

Communicating more effectively with our care team about what we want and expect from them, rather than what they want and expect from us, supports successful self-management.

MODERN CHALLENGES

Like it or not, we're in this together

MILLIONS OF PEOPLE live with chronic conditions in the United States, and many are considered preventable. As of 2020, the Centers for Disease Control and Prevention (CDC) reports that 60 percent of Americans live with one or more chronic conditions.[31]

Chronic disease is estimated to cost $5,300 per person each year.[32] To understand the scale and impact this has on the healthcare system, we could study the mall on a Saturday. Assume that 300 strangers cross your path during a one-hour stroll. For statistical purposes, let's assume that 6 in 10 of them have chronic conditions: multiply 180 people times $5,300 each, and you see that chronic disease costs your community alone $954,000 per year.

This was a small population to study in a short amount of time, but this visualization exercise helps us see a health crisis that's happening around us. Imagine how people with chronic conditions impact the health of the world both physically and financially. Imagine the impact on mental and emotional health as medical bills add up for a person with multiple conditions.

The combination of the costliest chronic diseases—diabetes, cardiovascular disease, and alcohol- and smoking-related health issues—contribute to the yearly cost of healthcare in the trillions.

As a community, why should we care?

A health problem afflicting 60 percent of the population is a problem for all of us. We are a collective community of people who generally care about our health. It is our job to help the people closest to us. The cost spreads to everyone, and not just in insurance premiums, but in the lack of time doctors have to treat patients and the months it takes to get scheduled with a specialist. Worst of all, we pay the highest price when we lose someone we care about and have to carry on wondering if things could have been different.

Everyone must chip in to improve the lives of people with chronic conditions. This can lead to uncomfortable conversations at the dinner table, but I encourage you to be the person who shows sincere concern, rather than the person who pretends not to notice.

How can we inspire our loved ones to adopt healthier habits?

- Show interest in their condition and allow space for them to express themselves.

- Ask about goals and barriers; show concern for their well-being without judgment.

- Ask permission before providing an opinion or offering solutions.

- Offer to assist with grocery shopping, cooking, or interpreting medical information.

- Lead by example; show that healthy habits are achievable and enrich quality of life.

Visualization Questions to Ask Yourself to Inspire Motivation

- If you woke up tomorrow in your ideal state of health, how would you feel?

- What one to three things do you need to change to feel this way?

- What would it take to maintain your ideal state of health?

- Who or what is at the core of your motivation to be healthy?

- To download a worksheet, visit https://www.lpnutritionconsulting.com.

Identifying the pathway toward healthy habits is an inside job determined by what you care most about. The answers to these questions reveal what you want, the primary changes you need to make, and who, or what, motivates you. See yourself as having the state of health you desire most, and live that life! Refuse to be satisfied until you become inspired by how taking action feels.

EATING WITH EYES OPEN

Connecting to your source of nourishment

I WASN'T RAISED VEGAN or vegetarian, but I did grow up understanding that family pets were my siblings. Cats, dogs, horses, brothers, Lauren—we were all Mom's children.

As young as I can remember, I got really upset when animals were hurt in movies. Hearing "It's not real" wasn't enough to make it okay. Then one day in second grade, my parents weren't there to cover my eyes, and I was scarred for life. I vividly remember crying in the dark as I sat petrified at my desk, alternating between my hands covering my eyes and my ears as the barn in *Black Beauty* burned.

Later that day, Mom called my teacher and hammered her with momma-bear grit for not recognizing that I had left the classroom for the nurse's office to call her, bawling my little eyes out.

My parents were careful to shield me from violence against animals, roadkill, and livestock farming. They knew I was a sensitive one, but they did not know, like most people don't know, what it takes to satisfy America's appetite. Or what actually happens to cute little farm animals. To protect myself, I learned to screen movies, but also to avoid knowing where food came from. The less I knew about the production of farming, or what unidentifiable food did to my body, the safer I was. This ignorance-is-bliss attitude carried into my adult years until I had the blood-drawn evidence that my A1c, thyroid, and cholesterol improved on a meatless diet.

Questions loomed as I examined hundreds of pages of nutrition articles related to chronic disease. Drawing correlations between type 2 diabetes, cancer, childhood nutrition, and the environmental impact on health rocked my sheltered world. I became acutely aware of how disconnected I was from what I ate and where it was from.

Not until I felt the difference in my digestion and saw the continual proof in my blood tests did I take the leap into the underworld of food. To fully understand the study of nutrition science, I needed exposure to animal agriculture.

This next part of my research would be nauseating, but my pursuit of knowledge always included two sides of the coin, and I needed to know the truth.

All it took was one video and a collection of images that I will never get out of my head.

Watching brutal atrocities committed inside the slaughterhouse felt like falling through thin ice. My whole body gasped in helpless pain followed by anger. *Why didn't the people shooting this video do anything about it? WHY?!* I took it a step further by reading a court report on a major pork supplier under investigation for multiple accounts of cruelty, and I felt sick for days.

My curious eyes couldn't look away, and my heart forced the truth. I couldn't help the animals, and I couldn't stop the abuse. It's the most helpless feeling on earth to know about violence against innocent beings and have no power to stop it.

All I could do was sit with horrified thoughts from images I couldn't release.

How does anyone in this world disregard the suffering of innocent creatures?

Why do we view farm animals as food without feelings but worship our domestic pets?

Why do we take our kids to the Miracle of Birth barn at the fair and then buy them corn dogs?

Aren't we better than this? How did it get this way?

Before I made an absolute decision that this was the only way animals are treated, I looked into what is considered humane slaughter.

Temple Grandin, a scientist of animal behavior and activist for the humane treatment of livestock, provided a general description. In a number of studies and demonstration videos, she explains her method of keeping cattle calm as they walk a long line between cattle guards that guide them into a factory. They saunter through, one in front of the other, toward a screen that shields each member of the herd. Behind that screen is a pressure gun they never see coming, and they die quickly when it's pressed to the top of their heads.

This is considered the humane way; raise them quick, move them slow, kill them fast.

So I asked myself if I could pull the trigger. Could I raise an animal to kill and eat?

Not a chance. Nor would I turn back on the health benefits that gave me a future.

The foundation of mass farm-animal processing is not hunting. It isn't part of nature. Nor is it considered healthy by an abundance of both anecdotal and evidence-based research.

Animal agriculture is a government-supported industry rooted in corruption, greed, and cruelty that takes no responsibility for adverse health effects tied to animal processing. The word *processing* is often used in place of *slaughter* because *slaughter* is a word associated with violence and massacre.

High-density confinement and rapid "processing" of animals keeps costs low and dismantles small-scale family farms. The faster and larger an animal grows, the better for mass production. And high demand results in low prices per pound. To accelerate the process, agrochemical companies like Monsanto were called on to develop genetically engineered bovine growth hormone to produce abnormally gigantic animals and increase milk production in dairy cows.

Chemicals injected into animals end up in consumers' bodies—

in addition to the hormones natural to the animal. After all, dairy is breast milk from another species.

In fact, dairy is known to contain bonding compounds within the protein casein that act like opiates on the human brain.[33] The compounds become concentrated in the processing of cheese, which has an addictive effect on humans. And the farming and fast-food industries definitely take full advantage of this.

I was horrified. The thought of synthetic hormones and addictive proteins linking to endocrinology disorders was beginning to hit me like a ton of bricks. Animal studies paid for by the beef, poultry, and dairy industries try to establish a "safe chemical intake" and state "no adverse effects" on humans, but I'm not willing to sign up as a subject to find out.

I began to feel very lucky that I had made the decision to stop eating meat when I did.

Many countries, including most of Europe and Canada, have banned bovine hormone, but in the United States, an overwhelmed Food and Drug Administration remains in the same place today as when the effort to ban animal growth hormones began in 1977.[34]

On the other hand, the United States Department of Agriculture is in charge of both creating the Dietary Guidelines for Americans—published every five years as the nation's leading source of nutrition recommendations—and the sale of agricultural products. This positions the USDA as an entity that talks out of both sides of its mouth, sending mixed messages to the public.

Twisting the Dietary Guidelines

The purpose of the Dietary Guidelines is to help people achieve and maintain good health throughout their lifespan.

According to the USDA, "It is developed for use by policymakers and nutrition and health professionals. Additional audiences who may use Dietary Guidelines information to develop programs, policies, and communication for the general public include businesses, schools, community groups, media, the food industry, and State and local governments."[35]

The guidelines are very specific about focusing on healthy eating patterns to reduce the risk of chronic disease by choosing nutrient-dense foods, limiting saturated fats, eating a variety of protein sources, and limiting processed meat. However, a wide range of statistics and studies designed to present specific evidence about Americans' eating habits is manipulated by industries that use the information to their benefit.

The North American Meat Institute (NAMI) shows us how they twist the guidelines to make misleading and blatant claims.[36] NAMI implies that Americans are *undereating* meat by citing *What We Eat in America, NHANES 2015–16*, a two-day memory-based dietary survey that allows researchers to explore relationships between nutrition and health status.[37] Based on the estimates of the National Health and Nutrition Examination Survey, NAMI claims that Americans do not overeat meat and that "just a small fraction of total meat and poultry consumption is processed meat" and "consumers are consuming meat and poultry at recommended levels."

The language in NAMI's fact sheet on nutrition has changed numerous times since they first wrote about their claims and false interpretation that "the 2015 Dietary Guidelines for Americans recommend eating 5.7 ounces of meat per day as part of a healthy, balanced diet."

To invalidate the claim that Americans are undereating meat, a study on the inadmissibility of *What We Eat in America* presents evidence that memory-based methods of assessment "are fundamentally and fatally flawed due to well-established scientific facts and analytic truths. . . . and [constitute] the greatest impediment to scientific progress in obesity and nutrition research."[38]

The guidelines are quoted correctly in *U.S. Trends in Food Availability and a Dietary Assessment of Loss-Adjusted Food Availability,*

1970–2014: "The *Guidelines* recommend Americans consume 5.5 oz-eq from the protein foods group (meat, poultry, fish, shellfish, eggs, nuts, seeds, and soy products) per person as part of a 2,000-calorie-per-day diet . . . According to the loss-adjusted food availability data, Americans consumed 7.1 oz-eq of meat, poultry, fish, eggs, and nuts per person per day in 2014 (i.e., not including legumes), *29 percent over the recommended amount of 5.5 oz-eq* [emphasis added]."[39]

It's important to observe that protein intake from dairy products and legumes is not included in this data; on average, Americans are likely consuming more than 7.1 ounces of protein daily from a range of sources. Also, not every person needs to eat 2,000 calories per day, which lowers overall protein needs. General protein recommendations vary per person based on weight and activity level, as dietary reference intakes range from 10 to 35 percent of total calories.

To calculate how much protein you need in a day, refer to page 190.

NAMI cites a 2008 article that states, according to the author's assessment, "new studies show meat can aid in weight loss by providing a sense of satisfaction that helps to control appetite and metabolize food more efficiently." Yet, in the fine print the authors have been compensated for various work in the industry by the National Dairy Council, Arla Foods, and the National Cattlemen's Beef Association.

The guidelines were recently under review for 2020–2025, as is the customary process every five years, and despite thousands of letters to the advisory committee, appealing to inform the public that dairy is no longer considered a health food—which Canada approved in 2019—*it was denied*.[40]

I would argue that if the general population were to slow their rate of sickness and disease by choosing to eat fewer animal products and more nutrient-dense plant foods, a great number of corporations would lose a lot of money. These billion-dollar industries would be inclined to fight tooth and nail to keep covering up the injustices they're getting away with. Yet, the evidence is right in front of our eyes, on our plates, and in our prescription bottles.

It appears that it isn't just Temple Grandin's cattle that are paraded along a conveyor belt while unaware of their pending doom. The only difference: farm animals aren't charged a copay for their drugs.

Metabolize This— Nutrition, Microbiome, and T1D

According to digestive health experts, "meat and efficient metabolism" is an oxymoron. The inside of our digestive tract—the microbiome—tells the truth about our metabolic abilities. A feature of healthy digestion is microbial diversity and its serving as our best defense against invading organisms. Damage to our microbiome is caused by environmental toxins, chemicals, and inflammatory foods. At the top of the list are processed meat, dairy, alcohol, and sugar, whereas the significant component to growing a diverse microbiome is in the production of anti-inflammatory short-chain fatty acids in the colon by the fermentation process of indigestible starch—*otherwise known as the incomparable badass we call fiber.*

People who live to be one hundred years old are known as centenarians. The highest concentration of these folks live in areas referred to as Blue Zones in various locations around the world.[41] Research demonstrates strong evidence of factors they have in common and specific foods that support healthy cellular function and longevity. The evidence also presents the importance of family, community, movement, and limiting stress, linking the holistic elements of our environment to physical and mental health.

To back up the value of short-chain fatty acids, we can refer to the diet of centenarians—high in plants, low in meat, dairy, and mental stress. A study that assessed the gut microbiota of individuals on a Mediterranean diet found a "significant association between consumption of a vegetable-based diet and increased levels of short chain fatty acids."[42]

Metabolic disorders and autoimmune diseases are linked to less diverse microbiota. This is specifically relevant to the onset of type 1 diabetes. An examination of studies on the relationship between microbiota, environmental factors, and T1D determined that microbial diversity provides protection against T1D onset,[43] while people living with T1D, among other autoimmune diseases, are found to have increased intestinal inflammation.

According to a 2020 study that examined changes in gut function, "Recent evidence strongly suggests that the intestinal microbiota plays a role in accelerating or preventing disease progression" of both T1D and Hashimoto's thyroiditis depending on the composition and function of the microbiome. Environmental factors have been determined to play a part in "the breakdown of host immune tolerance at the onset of both diseases."[44]

The evidence makes a strong argument for eating foods that build immunity by expanding the diversity of the microbiome while decreasing insulin resistance and lowering cholesterol. The same fiber-rich items on your grocery list can be used to not only decrease risk but also enhance health status at the same time!

Diverse yet balanced gut flora is the key to supporting a strong immune system. Though animal protein will contribute to diversity, it may also be counterproductive due to the health risks associated with inflammation as a precursor to cancer, heart disease, and autoimmune diseases.

Inflammation is what happens when your body tries to repair itself. A site of injury or infection triggers the immune system to respond by releasing cells to the area in need of repair. A long-term, or chronic, inflammatory state results from fat in the bloodstream, cigarette smoke, persistent high blood sugar, obesity, and the buildup of toxins.

Meat, dairy, and eggs contain precisely zero grams of fiber.

What Americans are actually eating is in plain view, coming on strong, and moving faster than a bullet train along the tracks of chronic disease. The foods Americans are *not* eating enough of could save lives, decrease healthcare costs, and improve quality of life.

The Dietary Guidelines state that fiber is a "nutrient of concern" going back at least three rounds of review, but the general population is getting nowhere fast as long as America and its influence on the world continues to buy in to the myth that more animal protein is better.

Conditioned to Fail

It's almost impossible to avoid food conditioning: the process of training people to eat a certain way. What we see advertised in large portions of high-fat, fried, and added-sugar meal deals may as well be invitations to the development or progression of chronic diseases.

By the way, our bodies are truly amazing at working through digestive adventures, toxins, and downright bad ideas, but just because we have the ability to eat almost anything *doesn't mean that we should.*

The combination of ads on billboards, television, radio, and podcasts on loop is designed to *keep us eating*, and networks have normalized overeating with shows like *Man v. Food* and wasteful challenges where the winner is the last one to regurgitate twelve days' worth of food.

Due to the dependence on animal ingredients in the Western diet, there's no question as to why more American people are living with obesity, diabetes, and heart disease compared to other modern countries. And while the cost of insurance and insulin increases, the US government provides billions of dollars to subsidize the meat and dairy industries to drive down cost, while less than 2 percent goes to the production of fruits and vegetables for human consumption.[45]

Kids are offered pizza, cheese sticks, milk, and cheeseburgers for school lunch, while fast-food companies advertise to all five senses with six-dollar meal deals that'll get you a bacon cheeseburger, large fries, soda, and a sundae. And when these kids become adults, the dietary supplement and pharmaceutical industries will be ready to receive them with open arms. And maybe, if they are diagnosed with type 1 or type 2 diabetes, they'll be offered a government-designed nutrition handout with the misleading message that zero-carb foods—meat, cheese, and eggs—are "free," until their blood work reveals otherwise. *Oh wait*—there's a pill for that.

Foods dripping in fat and sugar have become the foundation of the American diet, while preventive health education is nonexistent or inaccessible to many communities that need it most. As the rate of chronic disease increases, we throw money at costly tests and procedures that may temporarily relieve symptoms but do not address the underlying cause. This is one way people enter the healthcare system and never get out, as the perpetual cycle of tests, follow-up appointments, and bills never ceases.

Researching the animal-agriculture industry tied my guts in knots, but it was important for me to understand all sides of the issue. I started having nightmares and became irritable from a heavy heart. It took every ounce of self-control not to burst into a lecture wherever I went. School, family gatherings, at the grocery store—all

I saw were opportunities to make an impact. I had research to back up the changes in my health, but I was having an emotional reaction to the treatment of animals for food, and nobody else wanted to hear it.

These contradictions presented a moral dilemma that would determine my role as a health professional.

How will I work with people who do not share my values?

How am I going to explain the research without giving my personal account?

Can I protect my sanity and credibility as a plant-based dietitian?

Over the years, I have learned how to blend research into pertinent conversations specific to my audience. Recalling my history as a patient and the reasons for pursuing my career is a helpful grounding practice that aligns priorities. Presenting a teaching method that works with a wide variety of eaters is an ongoing challenge, but of the utmost value to advancing my skills. However, pushing an uninvited personal agenda is no way to make friends, nor would it be effective education.

Sometimes I work seven days a week to provide education to help people lower their cholesterol, decrease their risk for cancer, increase their insulin sensitivity, or reverse prediabetes. These conversations require knowledge about animal products. When we talk about meat portions, nutrient value, and fiber, each person makes a choice. They may choose to eat less meat, switch to plant-based milk, or cut back on eggs while increasing nutrient-rich foods at the same time. Each individual choice, as small as it may be, has a ripple effect on the whole planet. I can be satisfied that I've served my purpose when I help people make choices that contribute to the solution rather than the problem.

If I didn't have diabetes and understand how nutrition alters life, I might still be eating with my eyes closed. Diabetes is all-encompassing. There isn't just one thing that raises blood sugar, but a collection of elements in the environment that could affect us collectively: food, hormones, stress, DNA. Harm to other organs of our body can raise blood sugar as a stress response, affecting vascular health, circulation, and immunity. Cyclically, diabetes affects the entire system, and in turn, anything that happens in that system affects diabetes.

Five Ways to Increase Plant Protein While Decreasing Animal Protein

Go at your own pace.

1. Gradually replace meat with plant-based protein sources and meat substitutes. When selecting meat substitutes, choose based on the flavors you enjoy.

2. Where there is fiber, there is also protein in plant-based foods. Examples include black beans, chickpeas, tofu, quinoa, wild rice, oats, and pumpkin seeds. A variety of these foods will help to meet your protein needs as well as expand microbiome diversity.

3. Replace dairy products with soy-based and nut-based alternatives; milk, cheese, sour cream, cream cheese, and ice cream have plant-based comparable substitutes.

4. Explore the menus of plant-based restaurants and bookmark them for recipe ideas.

5. Take the brave step to learn about factory farming. You are a compassionate person, and you have the right to choose to eat with your eyes wide open. Accepting the truth about meat processing drives better choices.

Cashew Spread

The most versatile flavor that replaces dairy cheese.

- ¼ cup water

- ¼ cup fresh lime juice or key lime juice

- ½ cup nutritional yeast

- Handful of basil leaves

- 1 cup cashews

- 1 Tbsp dijon mustard

- 1 garlic clove

- Pinch of salt

1. Soak the cashews for at least 60 minutes to soften before blending.

2. Blend all ingredients together. (I blend half the ingredients at one time because I use a small bullet blender.)

3. Start with ¼ cup of water, and add small amounts of water or lime/lemon juice to desired thickness.

See the list of resources in the back of the book for some of my favorite sources for recipes and evidence-based information on plant-based eating.

Hormones, Autoimmunity, and the Environment

The growing incidence of endocrine disorders in the last two decades coincides with increased chemical production, and there is reason to believe these two things work hand in hand. The Endocrine Society, founded in 1916, recognizes that non-natural, exogenous chemicals, biological compounds used in the development of drugs and plastic, can affect the endocrine system. Among the society's members are leading experts on the health effects of endocrine disruptor chemicals (EDCs). They also partner with international organizations whose work is to implement safe chemical policies worldwide in support of a toxics-free future.

> The Endocrine Society defines an EDC as "an exogenous, non-natural chemical, or mixture of chemicals, that interferes with any aspect of hormone action."[46]

We are exposed to EDCs at home and in the air, food, water, soil, and human-populated areas in unavoidable quantities. It is estimated that over one thousand manufactured chemicals have endocrine-acting properties, and these are just the known chemicals. There are countless more suspected. Common examples of EDCs are pesticides, BPA, and phthalates found in personal care products. Consequently, measurements in body fluids and tissues show nearly 100 percent of humans have detectable levels.

The global production of plastics along with chemical-industry profits has increased to incomprehensible numbers since the 1930s. Yet questioning how these products change biology and lead to disease only began to hit us within the last twenty years.

The really scary part about EDCs in relation to autoimmunity is that *there is reason to suspect that pediatric endocrine disorders are linked to increased chemical production.*[47]

Chemicals of all sorts can alter our endocrine system depending on our individual sensitivities. For example, some individuals can eat nutrient-poor processed foods their entire lives without any ailments, while others have severe allergies and reactions of unknown origin. For broad reasons like this, chemical measurements that determine an amount considered safe or less toxic may not be satisfactory for everyone.

The immune system is constantly challenged to cope with our chemically dependent world. To complicate things further, as chemicals change and evolve, so do the cells of the human body. Hormone production changes as we age in parallel with the evolution of chemicals, leading to a variety of EDCs in already inflamed tissues. A complex intake of chemicals blended with environmental exposure across the lifespan makes pinpointing the cause for disease nearly impossible.

Endocrine glands are located throughout the cells of the body. Hormones are natural chemicals produced within these glands, and they have an important role within every organ in precise amounts that change as a person ages. Nutrition and hormonal responses have an important relationship to keep in good standing as they regulate hunger signaling, critical to reproductive function, growth, and brain development. Hormones are essential to survival and determine quality of life.

Minimizing Chemical Intake

- Locate a natural environment; head for the forest and breathe in the scent of grass and soil.

- Read labels on personal care products and be selective about what you put on your body.

- Choose plant-based ingredients free of phthalates and sold in natural, recycled materials.

- Avoid plastic bags at the mall and grocery store. Use cloth or a reusable tote.

- Avoid spraying your home and garden with pesticides that run off with rainwater.

- Cut back or eliminate animal products to prevent ingestion of hormones and chemicals.

- Use BPA-free water bottles, and avoid heating food in plastic containers.

NOTES

PART THREE

EXERCISE

EXERCISE KNOWLEDGE
Practical Methods for Movement

Physical activity and T1D at all levels of fitness

I HAVE A CONFESSION.

I cheated during the mile run in high school.

The run was part of a fitness challenge in volleyball practice. All my teammates had lapped me, and my legs hurt too much to complete the final lap around the track. I pretended to hold pace with a few other girls when I crossed the finish line and stopped, but the truth is, I had one more lap to go. I couldn't stand the thought of dragging my exasperated body across the finish line dead last.

The effort I made to get better at sports was undeniable, but I was the least respected player on the team because I was so unreliable. Every once in a while, I proved my worth by hitting the living snot out of a ball just because I was lucky enough to channel my frustration into focus. The same unreliability followed me to the softball team, where I occasionally surprised everyone with how hard I could hit a ball as an anger outlet. The internal turmoil was a solo mission and a lot to bear some days.

Clearly, team sports were wrong for me. *Can I blame diabetes for this?*

Kind of.

According to me, there was an "I" in team because no one else felt the physical pain that I did, or how it affected my mental health.

Back then, every attempt to manage blood sugar during exercise was an experiment with the same hypothesis: *If I overeat now, I won't go low during exercise.* I never considered the ramifications of playing with high blood sugar and certainly not that prolonged highs would cause blurred vision or muscles to cramp and spasm. The solution to my problem had been right in front of me the entire time, but I couldn't grasp the concept of exercising without overeating.

All I've ever wanted was to understand my body.

Fear cripples in mysterious ways. Physical activity was natural to me, but balancing blood sugar with aerobic exercise was like preparing to face a grizzly bear: intimidating, scary, and unpredictable.

I was so tired of staring in envy at girls who were physically fit and wishing that I was capable of being like them. And yes, it was about the superficial image of looking good, but internally, I was crippled by a lack of confidence and impatience. Why couldn't a few sit-ups and planks give me a flat stomach in the same amount of time it took to drop my blood sugar by two hundred points?

Diabetes was difficult, and I allowed it to determine my effort. Being told to exercise wasn't enough if I would never learn how to take care of myself while doing it.

A lack of confidence and criticism manifested from a constant state of fear during exercise. I always had a bag full of food nearby to treat lows, and if my blood sugar ran too high, my legs cramped so severely that I couldn't walk. I was either eating during practice or sitting out, feeling embarrassed in front of my team and humiliated by the coach who sidelined me. It was like losing the battle in a war against myself, and disheartening because I was athletic when I transferred my frustrations into power. At this time, there were no guiding resources outside of my parents that I could rely on. We got through it by packing extra food during tournaments and compression wrapping my hamstrings to deal with leg pain. From my perspective, "diabetes exercise specialist" was a myth, and answers were not going to reveal themselves out of thin air.

Motivation

I often hear people say they feel guilty about not exercising enough. Sometimes skipped workouts cascade into weeks without any physical movement, and that's when regret sets in. More often than not, we have the impression that it takes a high-heart-rate activity like boot camp or a big commitment like marathon training to get results. Some people have the type of personality where committing to something with an end point provides the jump-start they need. However, setting a goal based on a specific timeline can be intimidating for those who are not competitive and don't like attention while they work on physical fitness.

Routine and consistent movement are how we set the tone for what we want to achieve with our bodies, and we must enjoy it. This could start with walking the dog twice per day, taking the stairs instead of the elevator at work, or scheduling a few classes per week at the gym. These tasks become a basic need and so ingrained in daily habits that forgetting to do them will feel like leaving the house without shoes on. Exercise should not be torture or punishment, but it is something we need from an emotional place that helps us feel more focused, centered, and positive about ourselves.

What I have found most important about exercise is that we feel rewarded even before seeing any changes. Being present and enjoying the endorphins that exercise releases are primary to what might be happening to our appearance. Good feelings are instant. Physical changes take time. When we set our expectations on a physical trait by watching it evolve in the mirror, impatience can get the best of us, leading to failure or emotional meltdown when results don't come fast enough.

I've been there. Stuck in a rut. Expecting big results from very little effort.

Watching my body change through the teenage years was hard enough, but not understanding why I was gaining weight even while exercising daily was incredibly defeating. This was the perfect storm that led to self-consciousness and feeling ashamed of my body. I didn't know I had options, and some basic principles of exercise science would've given me hope.

Bad advice is just as disappointing as receiving no advice at all, and my care team didn't have the knowledge I needed. The goal was to exercise smarter and not harder, but underneath it all, I had to overcome the mental barriers holding me back. Once I became a dietitian and took interest in sports nutrition, I was positioned in the right place to find answers from reliable sources that provide priceless knowledge on how to partner exercise science with diabetes management.

Components of Exercise

An **athlete** is a person who is trained or skilled in sports or other forms of physical exercise requiring strength, agility, or stamina. *People with Type 1 Diabetes are all capable of being athletes.*

Exercise with T1D was a mystery to me until I became a dietetics student and used knowledge to stand up to diabetes. Facing challenges meant diving into the deep end and figuring out how to conquer my fears and misunderstandings, including those unrelated to exercise science.

I consider movement a daily practice, but I've learned that your mind rationalizes your purpose, your heart drives your desire to get it done, and your soul moves you toward enjoyment. These three components bond together as driving factors when it comes to exercise. When one is missing, exercise can feel like a chore we guilt ourselves into doing.

People who love to exercise often describe it as something they need as much as food and water. This concept is true for all of us because physical movement is one of life's basic necessities. The body-mind connection of movement is more than meets the eye.

Physical activity gives us purpose when we connect it to the bigger part of ourselves and fall in love with how it makes us feel.

The sense of meditation in motion works for some, but not everyone experiences a euphoric feeling after a hard workout. If you have a love-hate relationship with exercise, I have a few tricks up my sleeve to get you moving.

1. Take the air. When you have the kind of day that makes you want to eat chips and go to bed, please DON'T. Chips and bed delay the problem, but movement can help you seize the day! Walk away from a stressful environment by heading outside on a trail where your senses are stimulated by nature to change your perception. This can be a park or anywhere with green elements.

2. Find your sweat style. If you're bored with your workout, change it up! There are always other options. Keep exploring and you'll find a workout that meets your needs. YouTube has every form of movement you can imagine. Create a range of playlists that suit you; from weight training to tribal dance, there is space for everyone.

3. Music is everything. I have at least twenty-five playlists saved and titled for different reasons. I chose titles like "Rage" and "Energy" to match my mood and give myself an edge. There's a reason you see Olympians with their headphones on before they compete. It's called getting in the zone.

4. Check in with your personality. Are you a solo sweater or a group-oriented teammate? Connect with a community if you need an encouraging push. Make a group fitness class your Tuesday-night thing, or meet up with a running group that suits your level of fitness, or commit to a long daily walk with your dog as a fitness partner. There is a club for everything!

Physically active people with T1D are found to have an increased awareness of what they must do to stay safe while exercising. Fear of hypoglycemia during exercise is consistently reported as the main barrier to physical activity in a range of studies from the US to Australia to Europe.[48] And there's good reason to be concerned about lows; exercise can increase glucose uptake into cells by up to fifty times the normal rate![49] This indicates that we burn sugar much faster during aerobic exercise.

It is possible to exercise smarter and not harder without persistent low blood sugar or overeating carbohydrates. You must prioritize self-study to understand the way your body reacts during various physical activities. When you're ready to dig in your heels and commit to the learning process, you can begin by designing your own step-by-step protocol.

There are many benefits to exercise and diabetes! What does research say?

- Reduced heart disease risk

- Improved A1c and insulin sensitivity

- Reduced diabetes-related complications and risk of other chronic diseases

- Weight management

- Improved self-esteem and body image

- Friendship and community

Insulin Sensitivity versus Insulin Resistance

Insulin resistance occurs when our cells don't respond efficiently to insulin, causing a rise in blood sugar. The more resistant our cells are, the more insulin we need.

Insulin sensitivity occurs when cells uptake insulin efficiently and effectively lower blood sugar. The more sensitive our cells are, the less insulin we need.

Source: S.R. Colberg, R.J. Sigal, J.E. Yardley, M.C. Riddell, D.W. Dunstan, P.C. Dempsey, E.S. Horton, K. Castorino, and D.F. Tate, "Physical Activity/Exercise and Diabetes: A Position Statement of the American Diabetes Association," *Diabetes Care* 39 no. 11 (November 2016): 2065–79, https://doi.org/10.2337/dc16-1728.

EXERCISE PROTOCOL

Establishing your method of movement

THERE IS A special place in my heart where the dirt roads are perfect for trail hiking. I have always felt inspired surrounded by the mountains of Montana at the family cabin, and it was the best place to set out on another self-study adventure. After a few years of teaching indoor cycling classes every week, I was beginning to see the benefits of regular aerobic training. I had my blood sugars in solid order inside of a gym where I had total control. Now it was time to learn what it would take to manage blood sugar in the unpredictable outdoors.

I started by establishing an exercise protocol:

1. Choose a specific time to exercise two to three hours after eating a meal.
2. Test my blood sugar; eat fifteen to twenty grams of carbs if below 180.
3. Take fast-acting carbs with me in case my blood sugar drops unexpectedly.
4. Start on a specific route and turn back when it feels like I'm about halfway out of energy.
5. Tell Mom and Dad exactly where I'm going. This is Big Sky Country. It's a wild place!

Maintaining blood sugar was the priority. I wasn't going that far, but it looked like I was planning quite the expedition with a belt pack stuffed with glucose tabs, a granola bar, a glucose meter, and my license and phone. I felt a little ridiculous, but at least I was prepared.

With practice, I came to learn exactly what I need to take with me during outdoor excursions and how to decrease my chances of having low blood sugar. Also, I highly recommend using a continuous glucose monitor (CGM) to help establish trends and patterns in daily glucose levels. Low blood sugar during exercise rarely happens to me anymore now that I wear a CGM. This type of device is a must for an athlete, yet I have vowed to never leave home without fast-acting carbs, and I am convinced that the day I do will be the one and only time I knock on someone's door begging for juice.

Three Important Lessons

1. *Flexibility is a way of life.* Accept that blood sugar fluctuates. This is normal. Straight-line blood sugars 24/7 is not in the nature of the human body.

2. *Technology is incredibly insightful, but we are the ultimate decision-makers.* Pumps and CGMs are amazing tools for improving quality of life, but they can be inaccurate. If you suspect something is off or results are completely different than you expect, act wisely and safely. Call your care team or the device distributor or place a support ticket, and always verify an unusual CGM trend by testing with a blood sugar meter.

3. *Take care of all systems to take care of diabetes.* There is a wider world of physiology behind the scenes to consider as a total-system approach to healthy diabetes management. Our brain, heart, kidneys, and digestive tract work together with our endocrine system. Each is equally important to long-term quality of life with T1D.

Exercise challenges blood sugar management, but the benefits of establishing your exercise protocol will be worth it! Practice makes perfect, and a plan is necessary. Understanding how your insulin works under specific conditions supports good decision-making. Keep in mind: fluctuations happen, and every day is not likely to be exactly the same, but stay the course. Continue with your regimen, and be diligent in your exercise practice to balance blood sugar with healthy nutrition.

The greatest benefit to regular exercise is becoming a more trained athlete and using body fat for fuel rather than just glucose alone. Consistent effort decreases the element of surprise in blood sugar fluctuations as we study our patterns. Anytime we try something new physically, the greater the chance for low blood sugar and adrenaline spikes. Once we have a better grasp on the demands of physical activity, the more prepared we are to balance the variables.

Terms as they relate to exercise:

Aerobic exercise includes continuous movement at a more moderate heart rate. It improves insulin sensitivity, blood sugar variability, and cardiovascular fitness. Examples include jogging, cycling, rowing, swimming, dancing, hiking, and cross-country skiing.

Anaerobic exercise includes shorter bursts of energy output for speed and power. It supports strength, body composition, and lean body mass and can minimize the risk of hypoglycemia. Examples include sprints, climbing, HIIT, powerlifting, speed skating, squats, pull-ups, and box jumps.

Adrenaline is a hormone that, during anaerobic efforts, powers the heart to beat faster and increases blood flow to muscles. We feel this when we are under great stress and, in the case of exercise, making a hard physical effort. Blood sugar usually elevates under these conditions.

Basal rate insulin indicates a continuous supply of insulin that works around the clock to manage blood sugar, as insulin always must be available. During exercise, our muscle cells take up glucose as a fuel source, and insulin is the vehicle that makes sure glucose is present. If insulin is in short supply and blood sugar begins to run too high, the feelings of fatigue, dehydration, and loss of focus may set in.

Bolus insulin indicates a dose of fast-acting insulin taken just prior to eating or to correct high blood sugar. Fast-acting insulin typically peaks between ninety minutes and two hours. It's important to have a plan before the start of exercising to avoid having too much fast-acting insulin available, as this can be the cause for low blood sugar during exercise that may have a lasting effect.

Duration is a measurement of how long exercise lasts at any given intensity. If the plan is to maintain blood sugar during long aerobic efforts, insulin adjustments before, during, and after are critical to prevent drastic fluctuations and for proper recovery.

Glycogen is the storage form of glucose. Glycogen can be converted back to glucose to enter the bloodstream for cellular energy. Collectively, the liver, muscles, and brain store several thousands of calories of glycogen.

Intensity is a measurement of effort on heart rate. The more intense the effort is, the more likely that blood sugar will change rapidly. Short-duration anaerobic efforts often mix with aerobic exercise, increasing the overall intensity of the workout.

Personal Plan: Before, during, and after Exercise

The following is an example of what to think about when preparing to exercise and the factors to be aware of that affect blood sugar.

Type of exercise and duration:
cardio and weight training, fifty minutes

Example workout: 5:00 p.m. gym: thirty minutes of cycling + twenty minutes of weight training

Goal: Increase endurance capacity and ability to ride more miles.

Intensity

Thirty minutes of cycling at a steady state with brief hill climbing and sprinting intervals is an aerobic effort that includes high-intensity bursts when climbing or sprinting. Blood sugar levels are likely to decrease with aerobic activity but increase with hard anaerobic efforts. However, a **mixed workout** with aerobic and anaerobic activity can be ideal for stabilizing blood sugar.

Twenty minutes of weight training at higher repetitions and lower weight is an aerobic effort. However, lifting to fatigue or increasing the weight with explosive movements is an anaerobic effort. Blood sugar is more likely to trend at a fairly steady state or may elevate depending on muscular demand and adrenaline.

Before is about meal timing and determining the safest blood sugar range specific to you based on intensity and duration of your activity. Healthy blood sugar range is considered 70–180 mg/dL (milligrams per deciliter). Eat a balanced meal at least two hours prior to physical activity to prevent having fast-acting insulin (bolus) on board while exercising. Check your blood sugar within fifteen minutes of starting to exercise. If blood sugar is below 90, eat ten to twenty grams of fast-acting carbohydrates (without taking insulin) and wait to start until blood sugar has elevated; consider eating ten to fifteen grams with blood sugar up to 180 mg/dL if the activity will be aerobic. If blood sugar is high and climbing well out of range, be cautious about starting activity at the risk of developing blood ketones.[50]

Preferred fast-acting carbohydrates for exercise are small in portion and easy to digest (examples: banana, half a peanut butter sandwich, granola bar, Fig Newtons, fruit leather).

Considerations
A.) If you plan to eat within two hours before the start of activity, decrease your meal insulin by 25–75 percent for a thirty-minute or longer aerobic workout;[51] this allows blood sugar to steadily rise by the start of exercising so that additional carbohydrates are not needed at that time.

B.) If you ate within two hours before the start of activity and did not decrease your meal dose, the risk of hypoglycemia is greater; check blood sugar within fifteen minutes of starting to exercise. If blood sugar is in a healthy range, eat fifteen to twenty grams of carbohydrates to prevent dropping below range and check blood sugar halfway through your activity to determine if more carbohydrates are needed to maintain blood sugar.

During is about monitoring blood sugar fluctuations, especially if you are new to structured exercise or you are trying something different from your typical workout. Carry at least fifteen grams of fast-acting carbohydrates while exercising to treat a low on the spot. Drink water and avoid sports drinks unless you are aerobic for a long period of time, which requires a specific plan for nutrient replenishment.

Considerations
A.) Lows are more likely to happen when physical activity is new. When we try something that we aren't used to, blood sugar tends to be used for fuel at a faster rate. The goal during exercise is to become

physically trained from repetition to avoid low blood sugars and eating carbohydrates unnecessarily.

B.) Needing to eat fast-acting carbohydrates during aerobic activity depends on duration. In longer aerobic efforts lasting ninety minutes or more, glucose from food is often required to sustain energy output in addition to preventing lows. Sports supplements are also handy at this time.

After is about maintaining a healthy blood sugar range and fueling for recovery. The best practice is to eat a balanced meal soon after exercising for proper recovery and refueling.

Considerations

A.) To minimize post-workout high blood sugar that can result from the adrenaline factor of anaerobic efforts, cool down with low-intensity aerobic exercise. This could mean walking, slow pedaling, or any gentle movement for a minimum of 5–10 minutes. This strategy keeps muscle cells active just enough to continue using glucose for fuel. The last thing we want to do when adrenaline is on board is come to a sudden stop. Circulating insulin levels are low when sugar is used for rapid fuel. Stopping movement suddenly leaves glucose knocking on the cell door without a purpose or enough insulin to let it in.

B.) If blood sugar continues to spike out of range, indicating that a correction insulin dose is needed, be very careful with your dose. The safest approach is to take half the correction dose that is specific to your sliding scale.[52] The purpose of this conservative bolus is to correct blood sugar while accounting for the *insulin sensitivity* that exercise causes. Remember, fast-acting insulin can be active for up to three hours!

Pump Suspension and Basal Rate

- When choosing to suspend an insulin pump during exercise, limit suspension time to a maximum of sixty minutes. Immediate suspension can decrease the risk of lows while exercising but can increase the risk of prolonged high blood sugar after.

- Even when insulin delivery is suspended, blood sugar is still likely to lower at the start of exercising due to lag time in circulating insulin levels.

- For a workout of thirty minutes or more, consider reducing the basal rate sixty to ninety minutes before starting to exercise by 50–80 percent rather than suspending.

Mixed Workout and Cross-Training

Mixing aerobic exercise with resistance training has several benefits to performance enhancement as well as blood sugar control. Aerobic athletes already experience the blood sugar–lowering effect of steady-state exercise, but hypoglycemia can be a persistent challenge during and after activity. To improve blood sugar stability when active, resistance training before aerobic exercise has been shown to decrease the risk of low blood sugar.[53] Intense bursts of resistance efforts in an anaerobic state include lifting, pushing, pulling, jumping, and balancing.

The diagram on the next page demonstrates how blood sugar trends during aerobic, anaerobic, and combined exercise. Assume the dashed line is a blood sugar of 120 mg/dL, or 6.7 mmol/L (millimoles per liter), and the arrows moving outward demonstrate the predicted change in blood sugar based on that particular type of activity. A well-planned exercise protocol helps us to have the best blood sugar and performance outcomes.

	Aerobic	Mixed	Anaerobic
Glucose trends			
Main variables	Intensity and duration of exercise, insulin to glucagon ratio, fitness, nutrition, initial glucose concentration	Intensity and duration of exercise, insulin to glucagon ratio, counter-regulatory hormones, lactate concentration, fitness, nutrition, initial glucose concentration	Intensity and number of intervals, insulin concentration, counter-regulatory hormones, lactate concentration, fitness, nutrition, initial glucose concentration

Source: Riddell et al., "Exercise Management in Type 1 Diabetes: A Consensus Statement," *Lancet Diabetes and Endocrinology* 5, no. 5 (May 2017): 377–90.

Main variables impacting the way blood sugar responds to exercise:

- The amount of insulin in circulation

- Blood glucose value before exercise

- The nutritional composition of the meal or snack before exercise

- Intensity (how hard)

- Duration (how long)

- Weather conditions: heat, cold, and altitude

Design Your Own Protocol

To create a program that works for you, here are some things to address in your plan. What type of exercise will you do? At what time and for how long? Will it be aerobic, anaerobic, or mixed? What time will you eat a meal prior to your workout? Will you decrease your bolus or eat fast-acting carbs before exercising?

Answer these questions before you begin your workout:

- What is your blood sugar? Do you need to eat uncovered carbs before your workout?
- During your workout, what do you expect your blood sugar to do?
- After your workout, do you need to give yourself extra time to cool down? When do you plan to eat your next meal to support recovery and overnight blood sugar? Do you need to decrease your basal rate or set a temporary basal before bedtime?

For a worksheet to write out your plan, visit www. t1determination.com.

Elaine

This is a short story about my dear friend Elaine, who is one of a kind on the superhuman scale.

She is an avid hiker, equestrian, traveler, and mom of two with a PhD in equine genetics, and she has lived with type 1 diabetes since the age of five.

Elaine grew up with a love of running the hot desert terrain of Arizona. Although she was active, blood sugar control wasn't much of a priority in her youth. Like me, a time came when she had to face a fork in the road with a stern warning to get her act together, or life would become much harder. Fortunately, she stepped up to the challenge and became a brand-new, supercharged version of herself, raising a child as a single parent while putting herself through vet school. Indeed, this was no easy task, but I watched her complete her PhD with flying colors.

Of all these admirable traits, it's important to note that Elaine is a one-woman machine powered by Atomic Fireball candies, bananas, and peanut butter sandwiches. She took my indoor cycling classes every week for several years and never dropped the slightest hint of having T1D.

One day at the end of class, I walked through an accumulation of plastic wrappers surrounding her bike and asked, "What's up with this?"

She confessed with zero cares in the world, "Oh, I have type 1 diabetes, and I like Fireballs."

What kind of maniac eats Atomic Fireballs in the middle of spin class and doesn't let up in the slightest?!

Much to everyone's fear, Elaine is always the one who yells out "ONE MORE SONG" when everyone else in class is down to their last ounce of energy, including myself. Additionally, she's always after me to schedule a gut-busting ninety-minute class since the standard fifty-five minutes is never quite enough for her.

And she's always trying to get me to run stairs with her, but quite frankly, I'm afraid.

Needless to say, this gal keeps me on my toes and my heart rate pumping!

Every year since her son was very young, she's taken him hiking on his birthday. Now that he's a teen, he continues the family adventure by choosing the location. He once said to Elaine that she's too hard to keep up with unless she's carrying a forty-pound backpack. Just for fun, when her daughter was only two years old, Elaine strapped her into a carrier backpack and hiked the Grand Canyon. Five hours to hike down, seven hours to get out. No problem.

Most recently, Elaine scored major points in bold disobedience by hopping two stadium fences to run the stairs at Arizona State. Air temp: 100 degrees. She ran five sets of stairs five times each! It took about ninety minutes, which doesn't surprise me as it's her magic number.

As for her plan: oatmeal and fruit for breakfast a few hours prior with a conservative meal bolus to position her blood sugar around 120 at the start of her stair climb, prompting her to eat twenty grams of fast-acting glucose. She ate another twenty grams about halfway through, then completed the second half of her sets to finish with a blood sugar of 115.

She absolutely crushed her protocol with great results!

What can I say about this woman other than that I'm so lucky to be inspired by her?

Elaine is as real as rock 'n' roll. A woman with resolve and a badass, tough-as-nails attitude. She's sharp as a tack, she doesn't back down or give up, and she's got the sand to do what she puts her mind to. I'm also going to call her a supermom even if she doesn't like it. She'll make me pay up in ninety-minute classes.

What it takes to be like Elaine is prior planning and consistency with a dash of "Try to stop me."

MENTAL TOUGHNESS

Physical activity occurs between the ears

WHAT IS MENTAL toughness but a state that can be defined as a desire to do something so intensely that it borders on insanity? As one person jogs their first mile without stopping, another person hikes the two-thousand-mile Appalachian Trail. We are all different and choose our own physical and mental limits.

Lance Armstrong may be a scandalous cheater for doping during competition, but that doesn't change the fact that he won the Tour de France seven times (1999–2005). If you aren't familiar with Le Tour, here's the short and painful summary: it's twenty-one days of racing over two thousand miles on skinny tires through narrow roads ascending the French Alps in unforgiving rain, headwind, fog, and cobblestones. Taking harrowing descents on mountain roads without guardrails at fifty to sixty miles per hour and simply surviving doesn't make you a winner—just another hungry cyclist in one of the most dangerous races on the planet.

Although Lance was taking performance-enhancing drugs, no substance on the planet will pedal the French Alps on its own. Whatever your opinion is of the guy, he's still a warrior who did something beyond most people's wildest imaginations. He just happens to have a rather merciless and cutthroat relationship with competition.

What does cheating Lance have to do with badass Elaine?

Mental toughness is in the eye of the beholder, and it sets the cadence on life experiences. The willingness to get uncomfortable can lead to epic endeavors if we dare. Lance is an example of going too far to win, but a competitive approach doesn't have to be all or nothing for the rest of us mere mortals who don't qualify for the TDF.

As an avid reader of studies on endurance training, I find it fascinating that highly trained athletes have much in common with people living with T1D. It was this understanding that opened my eyes as to what people with diabetes are capable of prior to meeting the living proof that is Elaine.

When people with T1D understand how to leverage their regimen of insulin and blood sugar management with strategic nutrition, amazing things can happen. Similar to the day-in-and-day-out focus on balancing carbohydrates with insulin intake, athletes are ultrafocused on which nutrients produce the most desirable performance outcomes. For endurance athletes, this equates to glycogen storage and duration and intensity of training. These are the exact same components of safe and effective exercise that a person with T1D must understand, as they relate to their blood sugar and performance goals.

Endurance athletes eat carbohydrates to prolong performance and monitor their heart rate efficiency, while people with T1D also eat for performance, but also to prolong healthy blood sugar levels. They may also track how their heart rate coincides with blood sugar fluctuations.

Many people with T1D are disciplined athletes and exceptional at self-monitoring. Flexibility is paramount, and it's not easy to stay on top of all that is required to remain physically fit. Similar to athletes without diabetes, the mental component is just as vital as being physically capable, and perhaps the most challenging part of monitoring progress is what goes on between the ears.

Exercise and Mindset

While I was in the middle of my summer workout on a loop that starts with a 1.3-mile jog, stair repeats, side shuffles, and another 1.5- to 2-mile jog home, I chose to walk the final half mile. I told myself that walking was okay as long as I took the hilly route, but the next song on my playlist felt like an order to pick it up and start jogging NOW.

I talked myself into stopping again when the song was over, but a striking thought startled me; the message was evident and annoying, like a flick to the ear. I realized the power that my mind had over my body. Just before slowing my stride, the impulse of quitting fired down the back of my right leg and into my calf, where I've had cramping pain since I was a teen. My instinct was to quit because that was how I handled exercise when it got uncomfortable.

My blood sugar was fine, and my energy level was good. *Why was I giving up?*

My life's experiences flashed before me. The memories of quitting because my legs hurt and blaming diabetes took me back to the angry and defeated version of myself. *Shut up, calves!*

Although it wasn't my body that was quitting on me, it was my head trying to protect me with a warning: *Stop! You're in danger of being uncomfortable.* It took a split second to process what was happening from start to finish, but I shook it off and visualized myself jogging the rest of the way home.

You've done this before. Just. Keep. Going. Up that final hill.

And so, I made it.

I was never in danger, and my legs didn't hurt anymore.

I was soaked with sweat and painless pride when I got home on that ninety-seven-degree day in July, having realized the difference between being uncomfortable and being capable.

THERE IS POWER in the start—wherever you are in your

physical activity endeavors. Just press play. Your activity could be a one-mile walk or an eighty-mile bike ride. The first step to prep is in your head, as mindset is the thing that either stops us or inspires the get-up-and-go. Doubt can creep in at any time when we attempt challenging things. The beauty of exercise is that we don't have to go it alone, and we're guaranteed to feel more connected to our bodies as a result. We pull motivation to the surface in a number of ways: internally driven by reason, externally through community and friendship, or simply because we love movement and making progress.

I made the mistake of assuming I had plenty of muscle, until I hurt myself. I had never thoughtfully weight trained even though I was an indoor-cycling instructor. Why? Because I didn't know what to do and I was embarrassed about it. One day, I took the concrete stairs too fast with my arms full, slipped on an edge, went airborne, and landed on my tailbone. The next day, I leaned down to pick up Fluffy and pulled a muscle in my back that seized up my right leg.

Ridiculous! I'm too young for this, I thought.

I was hurting in several places and decided to try acupuncture. The doctor put me through a series of exercises to demonstrate that I had next to nothing for glute and hip strength, and my back would continue to be vulnerable to injury if I didn't do something about it. I also realized that I needed to work on my posture and core strength to protect my upper body—typical stubborn me, I had to hurt myself to understand what I was lacking. There was also visual evidence when the doctor took pictures of me as I attempted to squat. My form was crooked, I was leaning to one side, and my back was curved like a hook. *Not good.*

In order to remedy the problem, I had to develop a new practice.

The knowledge I acquired from the doctor was invaluable. Not only did I know why and where I needed to build strength, but I had a motive not to get hurt again. I joined a friend who helped me learn how to use the machines at the gym to strengthen specific muscles. As I built confidence in lifting weights, I found a trainer who designed a specific training plan with crystal clear instructions. I followed it precisely, and while others were sitting on benches, staring at their phones, I was lunging circles around them as I finished set after set.

Committing to this routine three to five days per week completely changed my body, and it wasn't a major sacrifice. In fact, the hours I aimlessly wasted between exercise machines shifted into productive time weight training. Most importantly, I enjoyed it, so I didn't slack. After a few months, my metabolism kicked into higher gear as a result of putting on more muscle. This led to better blood sugar control during and after workouts, as well as a fresh new exercise habit.

METABOLISM, CALORIES, AND PROTEIN

Powering the body with the right blend of fuel

W E ARE NOT so elementally different from every living thing around us that needs water, oxygen, and calories to survive. The average human body is composed of 50–65 percent water, held within our cells, blood, and muscles. The skin is our largest organ and needs hydration, while our brain uses 20 percent of the total number of calories our entire body needs for energy.[54] Powering the human body is quite the subconscious metabolic production!

Metabolism is an autonomous process that has one major job: keep the body alive for as long as possible. The complicated system of nutrient breakdown and rebuild known as the Krebs cycle occurs inside the mitochondria, aka the cellular powerhouse. For visual reference, take a look at a computer's motherboard. The inside of each of our trillions of cells looks similar to this. In fact, the Krebs cycle functions a lot like air traffic control to direct key pathways. The mitochondria are home to DNA and energy production—where food is turned into fuel. This is the process we think of as metabolism, and it's built to survive the worst conditions that we often bring upon ourselves by dieting.

It is scientifically proven that keeping our cells hydrated supports metabolism and organs to remain in standard working order, while dehydration provides an unhealthy environment where diseases can flourish. When a restrictive diet upsets the balance of our system, you can bet the first reaction is to either retain or lose fluid. If we don't eat enough, or we eat in a way that restricts important nutrients, our cells dehydrate. This commonly occurs from eating too much animal protein in place of a nutritionally diverse diet. Our bodies shed water weight in an effort to eliminate nitrogenous waste that is a byproduct of protein metabolism. This results from consuming more protein than our bodies can use at once.

The scale isn't lying when someone loses weight in a short amount of time by eating a high-protein diet, but we have to be clear about what kind of weight was lost. It's unlikely for an individual to lose substantial amounts of body fat rapidly without risking potentially irreversible cellular and metabolic damage. Our body recognizes the ingestion of large amounts of protein as a problem, and we cannot store protein for later use. The simple concept is *use it or lose it.*

Calories are units of energy that are used right away or stored as body fat for later use. This is different from protein, which breaks down to amino acids, which cannot be stored. If amino acids are not put to use within a few hours, the breakdown continues into ammonia and then to urea, the end product. *Urea* sure sounds like *urine*, doesn't it? Now you know how we get rid of excess amino acids.

More is not better—protein does not benefit the body beyond what can be used in a short period of time. Our metabolism is designed to get rid of what it cannot turn into energy or store. Amino acids are important—nine of the twenty required to function must be obtained from food. It may seem like the solution to building muscle is to consume as much protein as possible, but that's not the ideal method. The key to putting on muscle is equally about balancing calories, protein, carbohydrates, and fat.

Building muscle is a two-step process:

1. Eat an adequate amount of calories to build strength, and
2. Eat an adequate amount of macronutrients to maintain strength.

Maintaining strength and mass takes a variety of nutrients beyond the nutritional value of protein. Symptoms of an unbalanced, high-protein diet are irritability, mood swings, short temper, constipation, and poor energy—classic symptoms of inadequate carbohydrate intake.

Protein is the nutrient I most often see excessively consumed, with fat coming in a close second due to trends in dieting and misinformation about macronutrients. Although jacked dieting gurus may push high protein, it often leads to undesired weight gain, high cholesterol, and adverse health outcomes. The majority of weight-loss seekers that I've provided nutrition education to often have yo-yo dieting in common. Many have tried calorie-restricted, high-protein diet plans that lead to rapid weight loss. However, the plan is unsustainable long-term and yet, after the weight is gained back, they continue to overeat protein.

Each person has specific protein needs based on their health goals, desired body weight, and exercise habits. Knowing your individualized protein needs is invaluable information for long-term health, coupled with nutrient-rich, high-quality sources of protein.

Is there such a thing as too much protein?

YES, there sure is. There is no evidence that consuming more than two grams per kilogram of body weight has any advantage to strength because we simply cannot absorb more than what we will use. Sports-nutrition research recommends twenty to twenty-five grams of protein as the maximum amount necessary for efficient use at one time, so it's best to distribute protein rather evenly throughout the day. Since we don't store protein, like glucose, we can look at overeating protein as a waste of food and money. Protein needs are often greatly overestimated in the fitness industry and media. This misinformation is often led by paid protein-supplement advertising and ambassadors of products pushing the sale.

To understand your protein needs, start by calculating the amount that supports your goals.

Calculate Your Specific Protein Needs

1. *Using a calculator, type in your desired healthy body weight in pounds*; this could be your current weight, your goal weight after losing body fat, or your goal weight after gaining muscle.

2. *Divide this number by 2.2 to find your weight in kilograms.*

3. *Follow the information below for multiplying your weight in kilos by the recommended number that most closely describes your activity level.*

General Protein Guidelines (daily)

- 3–18 years: 0.9–1.0 g/kg

- 18–50 years: 0.8 g/kg

- 50+ years: 1.0 g/kg

Protein Needs Based on Activity Level

- 1.0 g/kg/day is a healthy baseline for a moderately active person doing low-impact cardio such as walking daily, short-distance cycling, basic yard work, or a part-time job on foot.

- 1.1–1.2 g/kg/day is for a person who is intentionally

active four to six hours per week. This might look like (1) one hour of cardio three to four times per week with light weight training; (2) thirty minutes of high-rep, low-weight training two to three times per week plus an active job on foot most of the day; (3) taking one to two intense classes per week, such as boot camp, TRX, or indoor cycling, plus additional body-weight exercises.

- 1.3–1.4 g/kg/day is for an athlete in regular high-level training. This could be an explosive-power athlete focused on aerobic or anaerobic gains and proper recovery. Examples: long-distance cycling, martial arts, speed skating, gymnastics, wrestling, or boxing.

- 1.5–1.8 g/kg/day is for an athlete in regular high-level training with increased intensity or hours of training. This could be an explosive-power athlete focused on aerobic or anaerobic gains and proper recovery. Examples: weight lifting, martial arts, speed skating, rowing, gymnastics, wrestling, swimming, or boxing.

- 1.8–2.0 g/kg/day is for high-level training that is perhaps temporary in intensity. For example, heavy weight lifting and training ten or more hours per week, focusing on major muscle building for competition purposes or part of athletic training for sports performance.

Research does not support any benefit from exceeding 2.0 g/kg/day, as this may negatively impact muscle gains due to dehydration.[55]

Conversions and Portion Sizes—*protein is almost everywhere!*

1 ounce of peanuts, almonds, or flax seeds: 6–7 grams

½ cup of cooked whole grains: 4–6 grams

1 cup of raw leafy greens: 3–6 grams

1 cup of cow or soy milk: 7–8 grams

3–4 ounces of steak, chicken, turkey, or fish: typically 20–25 grams

    (4 ounces fits in the palm of your hand)

1 egg: 5–7 grams

½ cup of beans: 6–8 grams

1 ounce of soy nuts: 10–12 grams

These values are typical ranges of common foods. Please read your labels or use a food scale for most reliable measurements.

The Mitochondria

You remember this little fella, right? Looks like a potato bug. The first time you were introduced was probably middle school biology class, when you had to draw a cell and all the organelles that live inside. If the "cellular powerhouse" sounds familiar, you know the mitochondria! There are a few fascinating and useful facts about this organelle that benefit a person with chronic disease: the more we have, the healthier we age; nutrition can help preserve them or accelerate dying off; and preserving healthy cellular function is key for people who self-regulate blood sugar.[56]

The cellular powerhouse is essential for aerobic metabolism, producing, storing, and transferring energy. This energy results from the breakdown of food. Imagine the periodic table of elements, with abbreviations like Na for sodium, K for potassium, and Mg for magnesium. These three micronutrients also happen to be electrolytes important for producing energy.

Eating a nutrient-rich diet is the best solution to supporting cellular energy and preservation. Our metabolism is the engine that knows exactly how to use chemical energy to keep us alive. Healthy, happy cells lead to healthy, happy aging.

Mitochondrial function is impaired in people with T1D. *Why?*

· Alteration in the cellular structure within skeletal muscle

· Fewer mitochondria due to accelerated aging of cells

Cellular structure and accelerated aging can result from prolonged high or low blood sugar, poor nutrient intake, malnutrition, smoking, and other unhealthy lifestyle choices.

Nutrition Choices that Support Cellular Function and Healthy Aging

- Whole grains

- Beans, legumes, and lentils

- Avocados, nuts, and seeds

- Leafy greens, vegetables, and fruits

- Organically grown foods from a backyard garden

- Low meat intake

My Favorite Super-Easy, Nutrient-Rich Meal

Check out my website to download the Fast Meals Formula.

The Mitochondria Bowl

- 2 cups of leafy greens

- ½ cup whole grains (basmati rice, wild rice, barley, quinoa, or couscous)

- ½ cup blend of soy beans and black beans

- 1–2 cups broccoli

- Salsa

- ½ avocado

- A pinch of green onion and sunflower seeds

- Sprinkle with flavors: cilantro, basil, sesame seeds, or lemon juice

Use this bowl as inspiration for creating six more similar meals to nourish your week.

Mix up whole grains by choosing basmati rice, wild rice, barley, quinoa, or couscous.

Try garbanzo or kidney beans instead of black beans, with 1 cup of diced sweet potato instead of whole grain.

Toss in veggies like cauliflower, bell peppers, pea pods, onions, and green beans. Sun-dried tomatoes with artichokes and capers add a delicious punch of flavor for a creative combo.

Mix up the flavor with low-sodium soy sauce, balsamic dressing, or low-sugar marinades. The possibilities are endless!

Remember this tip: where there's fiber, there's also protein. Plant-powered protein!

CARBOHYDRATE RESTRICTIONS IN ATHLETES

Energy must be in constant supply for optimal performance

THE MOST CONSISTENT evidence in favor of eating carbohydrates is the statement that glucose is our primary fuel source. Yet historically, this has not always aligned with the advice given to people with diabetes. Over time, I have struggled most to understand why general nutrition recommendations for people with diabetes conflict with national guidelines for healthy eating. Working as a dietitian brought up even more questions as to why many people living with diabetes are taught to treat all carbohydrates as equal when, in fact, they are not.

As evidenced by endurance athletes, there is a difference between foods consumed for fast-acting glucose and other forms of carbohydrates eaten during meals to replenish nutrients. A cyclist would not eat a high-fiber bean burrito during a three-hour ride but might choose a banana and a few sports gels. Tortillas, beans, bananas, and sports gels all contain carbohydrates, but they do not affect our blood sugar at the same rate.

The **glycemic index** is a reference that explains the rate of absorption of carbohydrates when ingested individually. However, we tend to eat carbohydrates in combination with other food groups, which can change the rate of glucose absorption. (For more on the GI, see page 110).

Carbohydrate metabolism during exercise depends on several

factors based on individual needs. It is advantageous to athletes to develop a timing strategy for both meals and eating during activity, when necessary. Consistent and measurable workouts help to determine the strategy by controlling the duration and intensity. When we practice the same workout at a consistent time, we can observe changes in blood sugar to help make better decisions with insulin and nutrition. Improving performance is a result of achieving the balance between insulin, nutrition, and healthy blood sugar. When carbohydrates are restricted, particularly in endurance athletes, inconsistent performance is a common observation. For athletes living with or without T1D, having low glycogen stores is a limitation that impairs training intensity over time.[57] Even if success is found while training on a diet that alternates low-carb with high-carb meals, the variation in carbohydrates can reduce the ability to adapt to increased training volume.

Research supports a nutrient-rich diet that meets calorie, vitamin, and mineral needs for all people, especially athletes of all ages, who require superior nutrition. Failure to meet their specific nutrient needs is detrimental to bone and brain health and particularly risky for growing children, who have high calorie needs.[58] Since we can be certain that glucose is the primary fuel for the body, we can also be certain that it's very important for athletes of all ages.

Determine your unique carbohydrate needs in grams, based on desired body weight.

- Carbohydrates make up 45–65 percent of total calories depending on energy output.

- Carbohydrates are for sustainable energy and replenishing glycogen.

- It is always important to take into account individual goals—i.e., weight loss, fitness, strength.

Carbohydrate Grams/Body Weight	Moderate Exercise (~1 Hour/Day)	Endurance Exercise (1–3 Hours/Day)	Extreme Exercise (>4 Hours/Day)
grams/pound	2.5–3.0	2.5–4.5	6–10
grams/kilogram	5–7	3.5–5.5	8–12

Source: Adapted from *Nancy Clark's Sports Nutrition Guidebook* 5th ed. (Champaign, IL: Human Kinetics, 2013).

Fasting, Performance, and Blood Sugar

There is very little research specific to athletes with T1D who train under carbohydrate restriction. However, fasted aerobic training in the morning has been found to stabilize blood sugar for people with T1D, but this comes with limitations. Fasted training in short duration at moderate intensity may shift the fuel source away from glucose and toward body fat. Okay, great! Let's walk uphill instead of jog.

Note this: if the intensity of fasted exercise increases your heart rate high enough, blood sugar may elevate.[59]

Dawn phenomenon happens to every human around sunrise, but people who measure their blood sugar understand it best. Hormones are timed with nature's alarm clock, the sun, and blood glucose rises as a result. This is a frustration for many people with T1D, but strategic insulin timing can make a positive difference in limiting the rate at which blood sugar rises. Experimenting with twenty to thirty minutes of mild to moderate aerobic activity after waking up may be beneficial for managing elevated morning glucose.

Personally, I have experimented with fasted morning cardio, and though research may support fat-burning efficiency with this type of workout, I find that it conflicts with meal-dose timing and the nature of my body. Many people with diabetes on daily injections take a basal dose of long-acting insulin in the morning. This may not be the ideal time to exercise, as the onset action time of this dose may take a few hours to reach full effect.

We might expect to see blood sugar slowly lower with aerobic exercise, but consider these factors:

1. When the next injection of long-acting insulin is due.
2. After fasting overnight, there is little insulin in circulation.
3. Long-acting insulin takes a few hours to take full effect after injecting—a delay in action time.
4. Blood sugar may elevate due to the delay in action time plus the effect of dawn phenomenon.

Ketosis and Athletic Performance

Ketosis can be simplified to a process of using fat for fuel. This is a highly spirited topic of metabolism, and although it is a natural process, a random search beginning with the letters k-e-t-o can lead to the most quacked-up nutrition advice on the internet. But it's important to understand both sides of the debate before meddling with metabolism, especially with T1D.

Very passionate ultralow-carb-diet followers aim to nearly eliminate carbohydrates in an attempt to maintain glucose control at similar levels as people without diabetes. They are highly disciplined and driven in their belief that carbohydrates are the enemy. However, living healthy with diabetes does not demand avoidance of carbohydrates, but rather finding flexibility in a nutrient-rich diet.

There is more to living healthy with diabetes than just A1c value. In my humble opinion, playing a game of "How low can I go?" with blood sugar values is asking for trouble, especially for an active person who needs to utilize glucose during activity and replenish glycogen. Maintaining blood sugar in a range that feels healthy depends on the individual, and we must consider what contributes most to a long, happy, and healthy life—*happy* being the operable word. Remember, taking care of diabetes is a holistic job, and every organ needs care in equal measure.

Ketosis occurs when glycogen is depleted, making fat, specifically ketones, the main energy source. This may sound like a great method for weight loss, but ketosis is an adaptation process that isn't designed for long-term use. Recall the importance of glucose for brain health and that we need it in energy reserves; ketosis kicks in while we are exercising and when we are fasting. The argument for ketosis explains that our bodies can adapt to functioning on ketones, but the risks are high. Endurance athletes rely on glycogen for duration and consistency. We can train ourselves to burn more fat by exercising consistently to improve endurance capacity. This will strengthen our heart rate. The consequences of driving glycogen stores too low increase the risk of low blood sugar and loss of muscular strength—a gamble that an athlete at any level with T1D should carefully consider before using the dietary-ketosis method for losing body fat.

Another risk of eating a very low-carb diet is nutrient deficiencies without extensive vitamin supplementation. If essential nutrients are not obtained through food, they must be supplemented. There is no guarantee that a person will absorb every vitamin and mineral required for cellular function through pills or powders alone, especially when the gut is saturated from a high-fat diet.

Let's not forget that vegetables and fruits contain carbohydrates. Eating a diet rich in nutrients is about being liberated from food rules and restrictions while having the energy to exceed physical-fitness goals and maintain healthy blood sugar levels.

Common Questions

Q: Can we train our bodies to run on only fat?
A: Our bodies burn a combination of sugar and fat all day long, while at rest and during exercise. As we become more efficient ath-

letes through consistent training, the body relies less on sugar and more on fat as it adapts to the workload. This is also known as heart rate efficiency.

When someone is not consuming enough glucose from carbohydrates in an attempt to use only body fat, you might notice exhaustion and inconsistency. When the body does not refuel with enough nutrients, metabolism settles into survival mode as we try to conserve every ounce of available glucose to prevent the breakdown of tissues. This is especially important for our brain, which only runs on glucose unless under starvation.

Q: Should athletes try the ketogenic diet or other very low-carbohydrate diets?

A: My responsibility is to provide recommendations about your health beyond the short term, based on research that supports positive long-term outcomes. Research may show advantages in short-term studies, but if the goal is to improve and sustain good form, the answer is firmly no. Inconsistency and unpredictability create an undesirable and unhealthy cycle that stresses metabolism and especially brain function. These stressors may have a negative impact on prolonged brain health and insulin needs.

Alzheimer's disease is sometimes referred to as type 3 diabetes because of insulin resistance. The brain requires glucose and insulin to help process information, especially while we are sleeping. When the brain is starved of glucose, it begins to use ketones in place of glucose for fuel. We can use ketones because our bodies are capable of producing another energy source as an act of survival. It's amazing that we can do this! However, this process can be described as controlled starvation. Simply put, restricting necessary nutrients is not ideal for maintaining a healthy body in the long run.

We cannot determine how long it takes for the ketogenic state to become detrimental to our brain and cardiovascular system, but we do know that its purpose is to decrease seizure activity in people with epilepsy by changing brain chemistry. To put it bluntly, please don't mess with your brain! Coincidentally, nutrition recommendations for delaying and preventing Alzheimer's is exactly the opposite of the ketogenic diet, which is mostly fat, moderate protein, and very low in carbohydrates. Additionally, the ketogenic diet is also the exact opposite of what most athletes need to perform optimally and consistently with proper recovery.

Q: Do carbs turn into fat?

A: Carbs and calories are not the same thing. Let's examine this:

Carbohydrates break down to glucose, which we constantly use for energy or store in our liver and muscles (a few thousand calories at a time). Glucose is our primary energy source, so it must always be available in the blood. *Calories* are units of energy that are metabolized as we begin to digest food. Overeating combined with inactivity results in excess calories that will be converted to triglycerides and stored in fat cells. Everything we eat has calories, so overeating even healthy foods can result in weight gain—when fat cells expand.

Q: I'm exercising a lot and I've cut way back on calories. Why am I gaining weight?

A: Metabolic confusion can result when we exercise too hard and take in too few calories. Evidence supports that food quality over total calories is a major factor in weight gain.

Example: eating only eight hundred calories per day is not enough for most people, but eating eight hundred calories in junk food can cause weight gain. Other factors to consider are poor sleep, inflammation, and stress levels, which can also cause our bodies to conserve calories and body fat. When low-calorie intake of poor-quality foods, high amounts of stress, or lack of sleep occur consistently, our body interprets a threat. The result is a slower metabolism to conserve energy for survival purposes. This can also lead to a higher risk of injury for athletes.

EMBRACE THE CONTRASTS

"You can't go back and make a new start, but you can start right now and make a brand-new ending."
—James Sherman

'VE OFTEN SAID that I hate snow because it's made my life hard.
Angry, impatient, and *fearful* are words I associate with long, icy winters. But yelling at the TV during the weather report doesn't serve my attitude. Winter becomes insignificant when I accept that the elements don't exist to ruin my day.

Even though the clearest blue days are often the coldest, the fresh powder sparkles with frigid beauty as the hard comes with the soft. This contrast supports one of the most valuable lessons I've learned in this life with T1D: *a change in perception is a change in attitude.*

Life with diabetes is full of contrasting ideas layered with burnout, anxiety, depression, and self-criticism. Describing diabetes as a burden, a battle, a fight, terrible, too hard, or something that sucks can change our beliefs. Especially when a person of influence is using these words. Pessimism can become the truth with constant association, while attitude is influenced by language. The way we think and the words we hear associated with diabetes tie into health outcomes.

Diabetes is a disease with the potential to elevate, renew, inspire, strengthen, educate, and connect. It is a personal challenge more often pushed back against than embraced. The tendency to self-judge and become hypercritical in an effort to protect ourselves is a natural defense. Comparing ourselves to others by focusing on what we may not have rather than what we do devalues our gifts.

Or perhaps we haven't discovered our gifts yet!

Living with disease isn't fair or easy, but our perception should not be chosen for us. Every person living with diabetes has the power to frame their future by practicing positive thinking. It is a skill that validates significance and purpose. There is no light without a little darkness; there is no ability to be of service to others without having been immersed in the worst of yourself. Using that darkness to become your best creates an energy that will precede you.

If you are living with T1D, make a promise to yourself that diabetes isn't above you or below you, but a part of you. And every day, you are going to step into the arena and embrace the experience.

245,000 hours.

By the time this book goes to print, I will have lived with T1D for more than 245,000 hours. A number this large is hard to comprehend because time is not tangible. Similar to untouchable time, the mind and body continue without skipping a beat, even for those who live with chronic disease.

Time represents change and evolution.

Time expects us to use it to become something—to evolve within ourselves, learn, and be curious. Our day-to-day lives are defined by choices and actions. We can choose a daily life of reactivity, or we can show up as if everywhere we go our favorite song is playing.

I've accepted T1D as a lifelong commitment, and I've maximized the potential of living a healthy life in partnership with the challenges that make me unique. It never crossed my mind that I could exceed expectations coming of age with a disease that was viewed by others as a sad situation. It wasn't just the hovering dark cloud of a healthcare system that set me up to fail, but the general attitude of disease management saying that it was a hopeless attempt to even try.

My rebel heart pounds the hardest at the thought of upgrading life with disease in the face of those who doubted me. But I forgive them, and I'm grateful for the position I've earned.

I am an evidence-based practitioner, which will never change, but what I am not is typical, standard, or ineffective. It simply was not my fate to sit back and wait for a cure while the spitfire inside of me was screaming to get out and help herself.

I can confidently say that if the American population were educated about nutrition down to a personal level and guided to make lifestyle changes as a primary intervention, the healthcare system would be vastly different. We would play offense as a society focused on prevention, personalization, and maintenance rather than masking our flaws or imperfections.

I can only imagine what that would do for mental health and happiness. And the ripple effect that would have on the world around us.

One of my favorite stories is *The Count of Monte Cristo*. It's a tale about a man who is handed an unfair life sentence but escapes to overcome betrayal while outsmarting his enemies in pursuit of the ultimate revenge. What he learns in the end is that revenge nearly drove him mad, until he realized what was most important in the new life he created.

This story resonates with both my history and my future of living with T1D.

If we spend our lives trying to reverse a negative experience, we may very well miss the opportunities before us to become better people. Living with challenges doesn't have to be a constant drag, but acceptance of flaws, adapting to change, and rolling with resistance can potentially create space for greatness. Growth comes from learning how to fail, while success is a result of turning setbacks into strengths.

Risk-taking, though it can be frightening, is a method of self-discovery. When we choose to swim with the tide and take an open-minded approach to living a different life than we expected, leaders and change makers blossom from that bud of new perception.

With the right attitude and a little fire in the belly, disease can't stop us.

Diabetes had no idea who it was messing with when it tried to take me down. I was angry, defiant, confused, and ashamed for a long time, until I realized that being diagnosed was my chance to live better.

I am everything about type 1 diabetes that people fear.

I am the highs and lows.

I am the imbalance of insulin and blood sugar.

I am what I eat, and that includes carbohydrates.

I wear the bruises and bloody spots from injections, and I am at risk for complications.

What makes me strong is owning my fear.

I have embraced my disease.

I never complain, blame myself, or get angry that diabetes chose me.

Add to that, *I am noncompliant.*

I am diabetes and I am ferocious.

I am willing to work with it.

I am willing to eat healthy and exercise so that I feel good about myself.

I am only as healthy as my attitude.

And attitude is everything.

Change your attitude, change your course in life.

To the diabadasses, T1D athletes, juice-box slammers, pump slingers, multidecade-diagnosed rock stars, affordable-insulin advocates, diabetes-education specialists in the making, YOU are diamonds in the rough. And you don't have to be perfectly polished to elevate your life's experience.

Prepare to write your own story.

Because all our experiences matter in improving life with diabetes.

And we have to make some noise if we want to be heard.

I hope you see that being healthy and happy is worth the effort.

I hope you're up for the challenge to do something you never thought you could.

I hope you're ready to accept the good with the bad and move forward without fear.

Embrace the time it will take, because you are not living an average life.

You're ready to rally and rock your playlist with a battle cry that screams, "I am the thunder!"

This is your time to show up, grab life by the beta cells, and declare your future.

Thank you for reading.

NOTES

BLOOD GLUCOSE CONVERSION CHART

1 mg/dL = 18 mmol/L

mg/dL	mmol/L
70	3.9
80	4.4
90	5.0
100	5.5
110	6.1
120	6.7
130	7.2
140	7.8
150	8.3
160	8.9
170	9.4
180	10.0
190	10.5
200	11.1
225	12.5
250	13.9
275	15.3
300	16.6

EDUCATIONAL AND MOTIVATIONAL RESOURCES

- **The Bean Institute:** https://beaninstitute.com/recipes/
- **Dairy-free with a focus on athletes:** https://switch4good.org
- **Forks Over Knives:** https://www.forksoverknives.com /recipes/
- **The *Game Changers* film and recipes:** https://gamechangersmovie.com
- **Lyfebulb:** https://lyfebulb.com/
- **Meatless Monday:** https://www.mondaycampaigns.org /meatless-monday
- **NutritionFacts.org video library:** https://nutritionfacts.org /videos/
- **Team Novo Nordisk:** https://www.teamnovonordisk.com/
- **TypeOneNation Summit, Juvenile Diabetes Research Foundation:** https://www.jdrf.org/chapter-finder/
- **21-Day Vegan Kickstart:** https://kickstart.pcrm.org/en

OUTRO

Cue the music, grab your sweat towel, and don't stop now that you're warmed up!

Here's what to do next:

Visit https://www.lpnutritionconsulting.com for downloads.

Contact me at Lauren@lpnutritionconsulting.com.

I'm a dynamic presenter, and I love providing nutrition education.

My presentations are tailored to audiences seeking to learn more about preventive health, exercise and nutrition for type 1 diabetes, language use in diabetes care, and plant-based nutrition for chronic disease. My past audiences include the Juvenile Diabetes Research Foundation, Association of Diabetes Care & Education Specialists, Children's Hospitals & Clinics, Twin Cities Veg Fest, primary care physicians, sleep-center specialists, and type 1 diabetes support groups.

ACKNOWLEDGMENTS

Thank you to the friends and family who encouraged me to write this thing. We did it! Gather up the dark chocolate peanut butter cups and uncork the Rebel Yell! A celebration is in order.

I have received emails from people all over the world who have a connection to type 1 diabetes, asking for my help or wanting to share a piece of their story with me. You all kept me going when I struggled to make sense of my thoughts or questioned the purpose of this book. We share something extraordinary, and I hope my experience has helped you embrace diabetes, elevate your health, and rise to your potential.

Mom, Dad, bros.

You didn't see this coming. I know. Being told to *make good decisions and come home smarter* almost every day worked! I wasn't always easy to be around, but I hope you are proud of who I've become. Anyone that knows us might say that we share some seriously tough family genetics in more ways than one. As the youngest, I've absorbed the best of each of you; that's a lot of goodness, grit, and ambition. Thank you for being my people and my safest place to land.

Tyler. You witnessed the entire transformation.

You made dinner for me, closed the refrigerator when I left it open, and cleaned up my coffee spills. You reminded me to shower, turn my sweater right-side out, and match my slippers while I worked nights and weekends exercising my fingers on this keyboard. You've listened to painful conversations with insurance, pharmacies, and suppliers as I stomped around the house speaking a foreign language about the inside job that the business of diabetes can be. You've smiled and pretended to know what I'm talking about when I ecstatically recite studies about the history of diabetes, exercise physiology, fiber, and insulin sensitivity. You've been my nutrition and exercise test subject so I can learn if the research applies to a natural athlete who has working beta cells. You've put up with years of temper tantrums, Saturday-morning playlists, and highs and lows, and still remember to replenish the juice-box supply.

I know a thousand ways to annoy you, but you still take real good care of me.

You're the handsomest, smartest, best cat dad EVER.

Thank you, tall boy. Love you.

Spin family. I'm sick with love for all of you! I wouldn't be here without all the laughs, gasps, and middle fingers you've graciously shared with me. Some songs will never be the same, nor the color red, whiskey, electronic bagpipes, or numbers between 85 and 115. Some of you have been close enough to follow this process with me. Thank you for listening and telling me to shut up and write like a fearless badass. If that's not love, I don't know what is.

Thank you to Kristin Jahnke and the Juvenile Diabetes Research Foundation for inviting me to speak with communities across the United States. I am honored to share the research on exercise and nutrition and to hear personal stories from the audience. It lights me up to have connected with so many people who live and breathe the mission to thrive with T1D.

Thank you to the AP Public Speaking teacher who scared the living hell out of me when I was eighteen. I'll never remember your name, but I see your black-swan, ballerina-esque image in the moments before every one of my presentations. There were only six of us in class, and you taught me that presenters don't read off note cards; they talk about what they know. And if I didn't know what I was talking about, I shouldn't be talking.

Thank you to Mike, my career development "professor," who taught me how to interview without apology. He worked full time as a headhunter and on the side as a helicopter pilot and international DJ. He would sit in a chair straight across from me wearing hot-orange cargo pants, electronic music playing in the background, while he fired off mock interview questions. It was a wonder how he could be fun and intimidating, extremely tan and focused, all at the same time. The skills I learned to 120 beats per minute explain a lot about my communication style and ability to multitask today.

To Team Novo Nordisk and the Changing Diabetes mission of ultimate scientific badassery. My life changed the day I watched the development team race up a notoriously fearsome hill in Stillwater, Minnesota. Thank you for your pioneering research, your eternally inspiring message, and for providing the living proof that T1D can be turned into a strength beyond expectations.

To Victoria Petelin, the best writing coach I could ask for, proving that two Leos do make a right. And the team at Wise Ink Creative Publishing for supporting a passion project that was bigger than my vocabulary. You all gave me the courage to let the words erupt from my soul. I'm an author because you believed my story needed to be heard. I feel like the coolest nutrition nerd in the world! Thank you.

NOTES

Going Mental

1 L.R. Rich, W. Haris, and A.M. Brown, "The Role of Brain Glycogen in Supporting Physiological Function," *Frontiers in Neuroscience* 13 (November 2019):1176, https://doi.org/10.3389/fnins.2019.01176.

2 Dean Sherzai and Ayesha Sherzai, *The Alzheimer's Solution: A Breakthrough Program to Prevent and Reverse the Symptoms of Cognitive Decline at Every Age* (New York: Harper Collins, 2017).

3 G. Riccardi, R. Giacco, and A.A. Rivellese, "Dietary Fat, Insulin Sensitivity and the Metabolic Syndrome," *Clinical Nutrition* 23 no. 4 (August 2004): 447–56, https://doi.org/10.1016/j.clnu.2004.02.006.

4 Sherzai and Sherzai, *Alzheimer's Solution.*

5 J.D. Gonzalvo, J. Hamm, S. Eaves, C.E. Muñoz, M. De Groot, F. Hill-Briggs, and R. Streisand, "A Practical Approach to Mental Health for the Diabetes Educator." *ADCES in Practice* 7 no. 2 (March 2019): 29–44, https://doi.org/10.1177/2325160319826929.

6 L.L. Liu, J.M. Lawrence, C. Davis, et al., "Prevalence of Overweight and Obesity in Youth with Diabetes in USA: The SEARCH for Diabetes in Youth Study," *Pediatric Diabetes* 11 no. 1 (2010): 4–11, https://doi.org/10.1111/j.1399-5448.2009.00519.x.

The Rebellion Begins

7 D.P. Zaharieva, and M.C. Riddell, "Caffeine and Glucose Homeostasis During Rest and Exercise in Diabetes Mellitus," *Applied Physiology Nutrition and Metabolism* 38 no. 8 (August 2013): 813–22, https://doi.org/10.1139/apnm-2012-0471.

8   Zaharieva and Riddell, "Caffeine and Glucose Homeostasis."

Shipwrecked on Diabetes Island

9   S.V. Bădescu et al., "The Association between Diabetes Mellitus and Depression," *Journal of Medicine and Life* 9 no. 2 (2016): 120–25.

The Cornerstones

10   N. Ramchandani, N. Way, G.D. Melkus, S. Sullivan-Bolyai, "Challenges to Diabetes Self-Management in Emerging Adults with Type 1 Diabetes," *Diabetes Educator* 45 no. 5 (2019):484–97, https://doi.org/10.1177/0145721719861349.

11   Eveline R. Goethals et al., "Healthcare Transition in Type 1 Diabetes: Perspectives of Diabetes Care and Education Specialists Caring for Young Adults." *Diabetes Educator* 46 no. 3 (2020): 252–60, https://doi.org/10.1177/0145721720918815.

12   J. Wiley, M. Westbrook, J. Long, J.R. Greenfield, R.O. Day, and J. Braithwaite, "Diabetes Education: The Experiences of Young Adults with Type 1 Diabetes," *Diabetes Therapy* 5 no. 1 2014): 299–321, https://doi.org/10.1007/s13300-014-0056-0.

13   A.E. Goebel-Fabbri, J. Fikkan, D.L. Franko, K. Pearson, B.J. Anderson, and K. Weinger, "Insulin Restriction and Associated Morbidity and Mortality in Women with Type 1 Diabetes," *Diabetes Care* 31 no. 3 (2008): 415–19, https://doi.org/10.2337/dc07-2026.

14   Orit Pinhas-Hamiel et al., "Eating Disorders in Adolescents with Type 1 Diabetes: Challenges in Diagnosis and Treatment," *World Journal of Diabetes* 6 no. 3 (2015): 517–26, https://doi.org/10.4239/wjd.v6.i3.517.

15   D. Russell-Jones and R. Khan, "Insulin-Associated Weight Gain in Diabetes—Causes, Effects and Coping Strategies," *Diabetes, Obesity and Metabolism* 9 no. 6 (November 2007): 799–812, https://doi.org/10.1111/j.1463-1326.2006.00686.x.

16   A. Caixás, C. Bashore, W. Nash, F. Pi-Sunyer, and B. La-

ferrère, "Insulin, Unlike Food Intake, Does Not Suppress Ghrelin in Human Subjects," *Journal of Clinical Endocrinology and Metabolism* 87 no. 4 (2002): 1902, https://doi.org/10.1210/jcem.87.4.8538; F. Chabot, A. Caron, M. Laplante, and D.H. St-Pierre, "Interrelationships between Ghrelin, Insulin and Glucose Homeostasis: Physiological Relevance," *World J Diabetes* 5 no. 3 (2014): 328–41, https://doi.org/10.4239/wjd.v5.i3.328.

17   American Diabetes Association, *American Diabetes Association Complete Guide to Diabetes: The Ultimate Home Reference from the Diabetes Experts*, 5th ed. (Alexandria, VA: American Diabetes Association, 2011).

Language and Attitude

18   J.K. Dickinson, S.J. Guzman, M.D. Maryniuk, C.A. O'Brian, J.K. Kadohiro, R.A. Jackson, N. D'Hondt, B. Montgomery, K.L. Close, and M.M. Funnell, "The Use of Language in Diabetes Care and Education," *Diabetes Educator* 43 no. 6 (December 2017): 551–64, https://doi.org/10.1177/0145721717735535; D.M. Zulman, M.C. Haverfield, J.G. Shaw, et al., "Practices to Foster Physician Presence and Connection With Patients in the Clinical Encounter," *JAMA* 323 no. 1 (2020): 70–81, https://doi.org/10.1001/jama.2019.19003; K.L. Roper, A.R. Thomas, L. Hieronymus, A. Brock, and J. Keck, "Patient and Clinician Perceptions of Prediabetes: A Mixed-Methods Primary Care Study," *Diabetes Educator* 45 no. 3 (June 2019): 302–14, https://doi.org/10.1177/0145721719845347; American Diabetes Association, "Standards of Medical Care in Diabetes—2020 Abridged for Primary Care Providers," *Clinical Diabetes* 38 no. 1 (January 2020): 10–38, https://doi.org/10.2337/cd20-as01.

19   Dickinson et al., "Use of Language."

20   Dickinson et al., "Use of Language."

Nutrition Knowledge: The Key to Prevention and Long-Term Health

21   B.J. Venn and T.J. Green, "Glycemic Index and Glycemic Load: Measurement Issues and Their Effect on Diet-Disease Relationships," *European Journal of Clinical Nutrition* 61 (December 2007):

S122–31, https://doi.org/10.1038/sj.ejcn.1602942.

22   US Department of Agriculture and US Department of Health and Human Services, *Dietary Guidelines for Americans, 2020–2025*, 9th ed. (Washington, DC: USDA, December 2020), https://DietaryGuidelines.gov.

23   Dean Sherzai and Ayesha Sherzai, *The Alzheimer's Solution: A Breakthrough Program to Prevent and Reverse the Symptoms of Cognitive Decline at Every Age*. New York: Harper Collins, 2017.

History of Nutrition in Diabetes

24   D. Lynn Loriaux, "Diabetes and the Ebers Papyrus: 1552 B.C.," *Endocrinologist* 16 no. 2 (March/April 2006): 55–56, https://doi.org/10.1097/01.ten.0000202534.83446.69.

25   K. Laios, M. Karamanou, Z. Saridaki, and G. Androutsos, "Aretaeus of Cappadocia and the First Description of Diabetes," *Hormones* 11 no. 1 (January–March 2012): 109–13, https://doi.org/10.1007/BF03401545.

26   B. Thomas, "Nutritional Advice for People with Diabetes: Past, Present, What Next?" *Practical Diabetes International* 21 no. 2 (2004): 69–72, https://doi.org/10.1002/pdi.591.

Fiber

27   C.L. Williams, "Importance of Dietary Fiber in Childhood," *Journal of the Academy of Nutrition and Dietetics* 95 no. 10 (October 1995): 1140–49 https://doi.org/10.1016/S0002-8223(95)00307-X; J.W. Anderson, P. Baird, R.H. Davis Jr., S. Ferreri, M. Knudtson, A. Koraym, V. Waters, and C.L. Williams, "Health Benefits of Dietary Fiber," *Nutrition Reviews* 67 no. 4 (April 2009): 188–205, https://doi.org/10.1111/j.1753-4887.2009.00189.x; S. Kranz, M. Brauchla, J.L. Slavin, and K.B. Miller, "What Do We Know about Dietary Fiber Intake in Children and Health? The Effects of Fiber Intake on Constipation, Obesity, and Diabetes in Children," *Advances in Nutrition* 3 no. 1 (January 2012): 47–53, https://doi.org/10.3945/an.111.001362; O. Oranta, K. Pahkala, S. Ruottinen, H. Niinikoski, H. Lagström, J.S. Viikari, A. Jula, B.M.

Loo, O. Simell, T. Rönnemaa, O.T. Raitakari, "Infancy-Onset Dietary Counseling of Low-Saturated-Fat Diet Improves Insulin Sensitivity in Healthy Adolescents 15–20 Years of Age: The Special Turku Coronary Risk Factor Intervention Project (STRIP) Study," *Diabetes Care* 36 no. 10 (October 2013): 2952–59, https://doi.org/10.2337/dc13-0361.

28   N.D. Barnard, J. Cohen, D.J. Jenkins, G. Turner-McGrievy, L. Gloede, A. Green, and H. Ferdowsian, "A Low-Fat Vegan Diet and a Conventional Diabetes Diet in the Treatment of Type 2 Diabetes: A Randomized, Controlled, 74-Wk Clinical Trial," *American Journal of Clinical Nutrition* 89 no. 5 (May 2009): 1588S–1596S, https://doi.org/10.3945/ajcn.2009.26736H; N.D. Barnard, A.I. Bush, A. Ceccarelli, J. Cooper, C.A. de Jager, K.I. Erickson, G. Fraser, S. Kesler, S.M. Levin, B. Lucey, M.C. Morris, and R. Squitti, "Dietary and Lifestyle Guidelines for the Prevention of Alzheimer's Disease," *Neurobiology of Aging* 35 no. S2 (September 2014): S74–S78, https://doi.org/10.1016/j.neurobiolaging.2014.03.033; D.J. Jenkins, L. Gloede, and A.A. Green, "Changes in Nutrient Intake and Dietary Quality among Participants with Type 2 Diabetes Following a Low-Fat Vegan Diet or a Conventional Diabetes Diet for 22 Weeks," *Journal of the Academy of Nutrition and Dietetics* 108 no. 10 (October 2008): 1636–45, https://doi.org/10.1016/j.jada.2008.07.015; J.W. Anderson and K. Ward, "High-Carbohydrate, High-Fiber Diets for Insulin-Treated Men with Diabetes Mellitus," *American Journal of Clinical Nutrition* 32 no. 11 (November 1979): 2312–21, https://doi.org/10.1093/ajcn/32.11.2312; M. Greger, "A Whole Food Plant-Based Diet Is Effective for Weight Loss: The Evidence," *American Journal of Lifestyle Medicine* 14 no. 5 (April 2020): 500–510, https://doi.org/10.1177/1559827620912400.

Fiber for Prevention

29   A.N. Reynolds, A.P. Akerman, and J. Mann, "Dietary Fibre and Whole Grains in Diabetes Management: Systematic Review and Meta-Analyses," *PLoS Medicine* 17 no. 3 (March 2020): e1003053, https://doi.org/10.1371/journal.pmed.1003053.

30   D. Aune, "Plant Foods, Antioxidant Biomarkers, and the Risk of Cardiovascular Disease, Cancer, and Mortality: A Review of the Evidence," *Advances in Nutrition* 10 no. S4 (2019): S404–S421, https://doi.org/10.1093/advances/nmz042.

Modern Challenges

31   Centers for Disease Control and Prevention, National Center for Chronic Disease Prevention and Health Promotion, https://www.cdc.gov/chronicdisease/index.htm.

32   W. Raghupathi and V. Raghupathi, "An Empirical Study of Chronic Diseases in the United States: A Visual Analytics Approach," *International Journal of Environmental Research and Public Health* 15 no. 3 (March 2018): 431, https://doi.org/10.3390/ijerph15030431.

Eating with Eyes Open

33   Neil Barnard, *The Cheese Trap: How Breaking a Surprising Addiction Will Help You Lose Weight, Gain Energy, and Get Healthy* (New York: Grand Central Publishing, 2017).

34   David Robinson Simon, *Meatonomics* (San Francisco: Red Wheel/Weiser, 2013), 59–62.

35   US Department of Health and Human Services and US Department of Agriculture, *2015–2020 Dietary Guidelines for Americans* 8th ed., (Washington, DC: USDA, 2015), https://health.gov/dietaryguidelines/2015/guidelines/.

36   "The United States Meat Industry at a Glance," North American Meat Institute, https://www.meatinstitute.org/index.php?ht=d/sp/i/47465/pid/47465.

37   US Department of Health and Human Services and US Department of Agriculture, *What We Eat in America, NHANES 2015–16. Centers for Disease Control and Prevention*, https://www.cdc.gov/nchs/nhanes/wweia.htm.

38   E. Archer, G. Pavela, and C.J. Lavie, "The Inadmissibility of What We Eat in America and NHANES Dietary Data in Nutrition and Obesity Research and the Scientific Formulation of National Dietary Guidelines," *Mayo Clinic Proceedings* 90 no. 7 (2015): 911–26, https://doi.org/10.1016/j.mayocp.2015.04.009.

39   J. Bentley, *U.S. Trends in Food Availability and a Dietary Assessment of Loss-Adjusted Food Availability, 1970–2014*, Economic Informa-

tion Bulletin 166 (Washington, DC: USDA, January 2017), 19, https://doi.org/10.22004/ag.econ.253947.

40   Health Canada, *Canada's Dietary Guidelines for Health Professionals and Policy Makers* (Ottawa, ON: Health Canada, 2019), https://food-guide.canada.ca/en/guidelines/.

Metabolize This—Nutrition, Microbiome, and T1D

41   J. Tan, C. McKenzie, M. Potamitis, A.N. Thorburn, C.R. Mackay, and L. Macia, "The Role of Short-Chain Fatty Acids in Health and Disease," *Advances in Immunology* 121 (2014): 91–119, https://doi.org/10.1016/B978-0-12-800100-4.00003-9; R.K. Singh, H.W. Chang, D. Yan, et al., "Influence of Diet on the Gut Microbiome and Implications for Human Health," *Journal of Translational Medicine* 15 no. 73 (2017), https://doi.org/10.1186/s12967-017-1175-y.

42   D. Buettner and S. Skemp, "Blue Zones: Lessons from the World's Longest Lived," *American Journal of Lifestyle Medicine* 10 no. 5 (July 2016): 318–21, https://doi.org/10.1177/1559827616637066; S. Vasto, C. Rizzo, and C. Caruso, "Centenarians and Diet: What They Eat in the Western Part of Sicily," *Immunity and Ageing* 9 no. 10 (2012), https://doi.org/10.1186/1742-4933-9-10.

42   F. De Filippis, N. Pellegrini, L. Vannini, I.B. Jeffery, A. La Storia, L. Laghi, D.I. Serrazanetti, R. Di Cagno, I. Ferrocino, C. Lazzi, S. Turroni, L. Cocolin, P. Brigidi, E. Neviani, M. Gobbetti, P.W. O'Toole, D. Ercolini, "High-Level Adherence to a Mediterranean Diet Beneficially Impacts the Gut Microbiota and Associated Metabolome," *Gut* 65 no. 11 (November 2016): 1812–21, https://doi.org/10.1136/gutjnl-2015-309957.

43   S. Dedrick, B. Sundaresh, Q. Huang, et al., "The Role of Gut Microbiota and Environmental Factors in Type 1 Diabetes Pathogenesis," *Frontiers in Endocrinology* 11 (2020): 78, https://doi.org/10.3389/fendo.2020.00078; P.G. Gavin, J.A. Mullaney, D. Loo, K.L. Cao, P.A. Gottlieb, M.M. Hill, D. Zipris, and E.E. Hamilton-Williams, "Intestinal Metaproteomics Reveals Host-Microbiota Interactions in Subjects at Risk for Type 1 Diabetes," *Diabetes Care* 41 no. 10 (October 2018): 2178–86, https://doi.org/10.2337/dc18-0777.

44   A.C. Fenneman, E. Rampanelli, Y.S. Yin, J. Ames, M.J. Blaser, E. Fliers, and M. Nieuwdorp, "Gut Microbiota and Metabolites in the Pathogenesis of Endocrine Disease," *Biochemical Society Transactions* 48 no. 3 (June 2020): 915–31, https://doi.org/10.1042/BST20190686.

45   Robinson Simon, *Meatonomics*, 79.

46   Endocrine Society (2014). *Introduction to Endocrine Disrupting Chemicals (EDCs) A guide for Public Interest Organizations and Policy-Makers.* https://www.endocrine.org/-/media/endosociety/files/advocacy-and-outreach/important-documents/introduction-to-endocrine-disrupting-chemicals.pdf.

47   J.D. Meeker, "Exposure to Environmental Endocrine Disruptors and Child Development," *Archives of Pediatrics and Adolescent Medicine* 166 no. 10 (2012): 952–58, https://doi.org/10.1001/archpediatrics.2012.241.

Exercise Knowledge: Practical Methods for Movement

48   B. Bohn, A. Herbst, M. Pfeifer, D. Krakow, S. Zimny, F. Kopp, A. Melmer, J.M. Steinacker, and R.W. Holl, "Impact of Physical Activity on Glycemic Control and Prevalence of Cardiovascular Risk Factors in Adults With Type 1 Diabetes: A Cross-Sectional Multicenter Study of 18,028 Patients," *Diabetes Care* 38 no. 8 (August 2015) 1536–43, https://doi.org/10.2337/dc15-0030.

49   L. Sylow, M. Kleinert, E. Richter, et al., "Exercise-Stimulated Glucose Uptake—Regulation and Implications for Glycaemic Control," *Nature Reviews Endocrinology* 13 (2017), 133–48, https://doi.org/10.1038/nrendo.2016.162.

Exercise Protocol

50   M.C. Riddell, I.W. Gallen, C.E. Smart, C.E. Taplin, P. Adolfsson, A.N. Lumb, A. Kowalski, R. Rabasa-Lhoret, R.J. McCrimmon, C. Hume, F. Annan, P.A. Fournier, C. Graham, B. Bode, P. Galassetti, T.W. Jones, I.S. Millán, T. Heise, A.L. Peters, A. Petz, and L.M. Laffel, "Exercise Management in Type 1 Diabetes: A Consensus Statement," *Lancet Diabetes and Endocrinology* 5 no. 5 (May 2017): 377–90, https://

doi.org/10.1016/S2213-8587(17)30014-1.

51   Riddell et al., "Exercise Management."

52   S.R. Colberg, R.J. Sigal, J.E. Yardley, M.C. Riddell, D.W. Dunstan, P.C. Dempsey, E.S. Horton, K. Castorino, and D.F. Tate, "Physical Activity/Exercise and Diabetes: A Position Statement of the American Diabetes Association," *Diabetes Care* 39 no. 11 (November 2016): 2065–79, https://doi.org/10.2337/dc16-1728.

53   J.E. Yardley, G.P. Kenny, B.A. Perkins, M.C. Riddell, J. Malcolm, P. Boulay, F. Khandwala, and R.J. Sigal, "Effects of Performing Resistance Exercise Before Versus After Aerobic Exercise on Glycemia in Type 1 Diabetes," *Diabetes Care* 35 no. 4 (April 2012): 669–75, https://doi.org/10.2337/dc11-1844.

Mental Toughness

54   L.R. Rich, W. Harris, and A.M. Brown, "The Role of Brain Glycogen in Supporting Physiological Function," *Frontiers in Neuroscience* 13 (2019): 1176, https://doi.org/10.3389/fnins.2019.01176.

55   Nancy Clark, *Nancy Clark's Sports Nutrition Guidebook* 5th ed. (Champaign, IL: Human Kinetics, 2013).

56   C.M.F. Monaco, M.C. Hughes, S.V. Ramos, N.E. Varah, C. Lamberz, F.A. Rahman, C. McGlory, M.A. Tarnopolsky, M.P. Krause, R. Laham, T.J. Hawke, and C.G.R. Perry, "Altered Mitochondrial Bioenergetics and Ultrastructure in the Skeletal Muscle of Young Adults with Type 1 Diabetes," *Diabetologia* 61 no. 6 (June 2018): 1411–23, https://doi.org/10.1007/s00125-018-4602-6.

Carbohydrate Restriction in Athletes

57   J.D. Bartlett, J.A. Hawley, and J.P. Morton, "Carbohydrate Availability and Exercise Training Adaptation: Too Much of a Good Thing?" *European Journal of Sport Science* 15 no. 1 (2015): 3–12, https://doi.org/10.1080/17461391.2014.920926.

58   C.E. Smart, F. Annan, L.P. Bruno, L.A. Higgins, and C.L.

Acerini, "Nutritional Management in Children and Adolescents with Diabetes," *Pediatric Diabetes* 15 no. S20 (2014): 135–53.

59   S. Scott, P. Kempf, L. Bally, and C. Stettler, "Carbohydrate Intake in the Context of Exercise in People with Type 1 Diabetes," *Nutrients* 11 no. 12 (December 2019): 3017, https://doi.org/10.3390/nu11123017.